Infection Prevention and Control Issues in the Environment of Care®

Second Edition

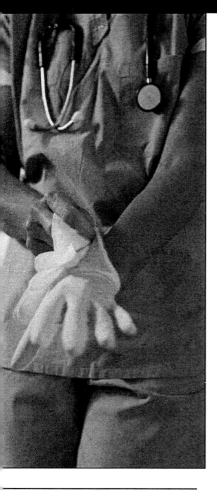

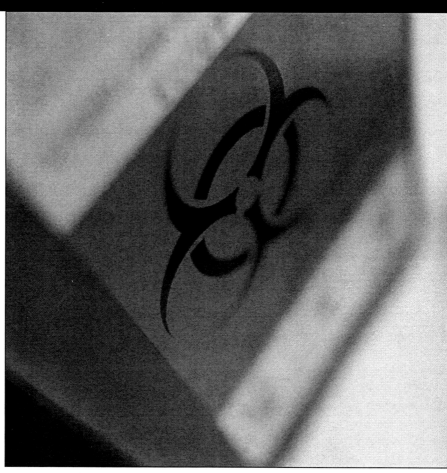

Joint Commission
Resources

Senior Editor: Ilese J. Chatman

Project Manager: Meghan Anderson

Publications Manager: Paul Reis

Associate Director, Production: Johanna Harris

Associate Director, Editorial Development: Diane Bell

Executive Director: Catherine Chopp Hinckley, Ph.D.

Joint Commission/JCR Reviewers: John Fishbeck, Kelly Fugate, Jerry Gervais, Louise Kuhny, Susan Slavish, Barbara Soule, Diane Bell, Catherine Hinckley, Paul Reis

Joint Commission Resources Mission

The mission of Joint Commission Resources (JCR) is to continuously improve the safety and quality of health care in the United States and in the international community through the provision of education, publications, consultation, and evaluation services.

Joint Commission Resources educational programs and publications support, but are separate from, the accreditation activities of The Joint Commission. Attendees at Joint Commission Resources educational programs and purchasers of Joint Commission Resources publications receive no special consideration or treatment in, or confidential information about, the accreditation process.

The inclusion of an organization name, product, or service in a Joint Commission Resources publication should not be construed as an endorsement of such organization, product, or service, nor is failure to include an organization name, product, or service to be construed as disapproval.

Printed in the U.S.A. 5 4 3 2 1

Requests for permission to make copies of any part of this work should be mailed to
Permissions Editor
Department of Publications
Joint Commission Resources
One Renaissance Boulevard
Oakbrook Terrace, Illinois 60181
permissions@jcrinc.com

ISBN: 978-1-59940-303-8
Library of Congress Control Number: 2009925542

For more information about Joint Commission Resources, please visit http://www.jcrinc.com.

Table of Contents

Chapter 3: Equipment

Chapter 4: Environmental Services

Chapter 5: Utilities

Introduction

The data are impossible to ignore. More than 2 million health care–associated infections (HAIs) are reported annually in the United States, resulting in more than 100,000 inpatient deaths and an estimated $30.5 billion in additional health care costs, according to the Centers for Disease Control and Prevention (CDC).[1] As many as 1.4 million cases of HAI occur globally at any given time.[2] That was the case in 2005 when the first edition of *Infection Control Issues in the Environment of Care* was published, and all indications are that these rates have not changed.

But change is needed. The Centers for Medicare & Medicaid Services (CMS) announced that it will no longer reimburse for extra costs associated with certain types of HAIs (*see* Sidebar I-1, right) acquired while the patient was receiving care, giving hospitals and health care facilities even more incentive to implement prevention measures.[3] In addition, although Legionnaires' disease is not currently included in the hospital-acquired conditions (HAC) list (check the CMS Web site at http://www.cms.hhs.gov for further updates regarding the inclusion of this disease to the list), the CMS included 10 categories of conditions that were selected for the HAC payment provision. Payment implications for these 10 categories of HACs began October 1, 2008.

Although hospitals and other health care organizations heighten prevention efforts and control the acquisition and transmission of such infections, they are being stymied by a growing list of contributing factors that, to a large extent, seem to be beyond their control. Increasing numbers of patients with compromised immune systems, technology that improves medical outcomes but introduces more complicated procedures, staff shortages, the appearance of new infectious organisms just as the old enemies gain resistance, and the need to constantly renovate and construct new facilities continue to grow.

Sidebar I-1: The 10 Categories of Hospital-Acquired Conditions

1. Foreign Object Retained After Surgery
2. Air Embolism
3. Blood Incompatibility
4. Stage III and IV Pressure Ulcers
5. Falls and Trauma
   - Fractures
   - Dislocations
   - Intracranial Injuries
   - Crushing Injuries
   - Burns
   - Electric Shock
6. Manifestations of Poor Glycemic Control
   - Diabetic Ketoacidosis
   - Nonketotic Hyperosmolar Coma
   - Hypoglycemic Coma
   - Secondary Diabetes with Ketoacidosis
   - Secondary Diabetes with Hyperosmolarity
7. Catheter-Associated Urinary Tract Infection
8. Vascular Catheter-Associated Infection
9. Surgical Site Infection following:
   - Coronary Artery Bypass Graft—Mediastinitis
   - Bariatric Surgery
     - Laparoscopic Gastric Bypass
     - Gastroenterostomy
     - Laparoscopic Gastric Restrictive Surgery
   - Orthopedic Procedures
     - Spine
     - Neck
     - Shoulder
     - Elbow
10. Deep Vein Thrombosis/Pulmonary Embolism
    - Total Knee Replacement
    - Hip Replacement

The Connection Between Infection and the Physical Environment

Infection preventionists and hospital epidemiologists are gaining on the microbes, using tactics and strategies honed in the field. Environment of care (EC) professionals remain important allies. It is true that effective management of the EC, or the organization's physical environment, is not the most critical element in the fight against HAIs. The vast majority of infections are transmitted by personal contact abetted by poor hygiene habits—primarily the simple failure of staff and licensed independent practitioners to wash their hands. For this reason, the overwhelming majority of resources available on infection prevention and control (IC) take up EC issues fleetingly, if at all.

However, IC and EC are linked in today's critical access hospitals, hospitals, long term care organizations, and other health care settings. Some of these links include, but are not limited to, the following EC issues:

- Routine housekeeping
- Sterilization of medical devices
- Containment of contaminated laundry
- Installation and maintenance of filters to trap airborne contaminants in the air
- Selection and care of toys in the pediatric unit
- Treatment of water used for dialysis
- Use of standard precautions by plumbers and electricians
- Use of tacky mats or other dust-control devices at the exits of construction zones
- Placement of hand-washing sinks, hand rub dispensers, and hygiene products
- Cleaning carpets

Aspergillus species and *Legionella* species, two of the most well known organisms causing HAIs, attack through the most basic components of the environment—the air and water. Failures in one or more facets of the physical environment—ventilation systems, water systems, or inadequate cleaning processes—can result in death and costly illnesses.

The Joint Commission standards and requirements, including the EC and IC standards, insist on the connection. They require organizations to monitor, analyze, and improve conditions in the environment, specifically including IC. And to a much greater degree than ever before, the requirements insist that organization leadership assume responsibility for reducing the risk and transmission of HAIs, including environmental risks. These standards and requirements place accountability for the effectiveness of an organization's IC program squarely with its leaders, who are responsible for assuring adequate staff training in the IC, communicating and coordinating efforts with the health department and other community agencies, and allocating sufficient resources to support the program.

Ongoing risk assessment and monitoring that feature meaningful performance measurement are called for—the historical emphasis on surveillance is now supplemented by an emphasis on timely intervention, data collection, and data analysis.

Inside This New Edition

This new edition is designed to help infection preventionists and EC professionals to collaborate on issues surrounding the EC to develop programs that will protect patients, employees, visitors, and other staff from HAIs. This edition explores various issues and concerns in EC with IC (lethal and otherwise) that can be prevented through proper management of the EC in the following areas:

- Construction and renovation
- Emergency management
- Environmental services
- Hand hygiene
- Infectious materials and waste
- Medical equipment
- Utilities

Chapter 1, "Making the Connection: Infection Prevention and Control and Environment of Care Issues," discusses the newly revised IC– and EC–related standards, as well as other aspects of The Joint Commission's commitment to IC issues. It defines the connection between IC and EC standards and emphasizes the importance of collaboration between IC and EC professionals. Chapter 1 examines IC as a Priority Focus Area, describes the on-site physical environment activities as preventive tools, explains the role of the infection preventionist, and looks at issues in the public reporting of HAIs.

Chapter 2, "Human Factors for Infection Prevention and Control and Environment of Care Professionals," delves deeper into the working partnership between IC and EC employees, discusses education and training, and provides information on the issue of hand hygiene, including placement of hand rub dispensers. The CDC and the World Health Organization (WHO) guidelines are also discussed.

Chapter 3, "Equipment," discusses various aspects and accountabilities related to IC issues, such as cleaning methods, biomedical engineering, reusable equipment, and centralized processing.

Chapter 4, "Environmental Services," examines issues related to maintaining the physical environment and IC, such as housekeeping and regulated medical waste disposal, based on guidelines developed by the CDC and WHO.

Chapter 5, "Utilities," discusses the heart of the IC/EC connection—IC issues such as air handling, ventilation, and water distribution systems (including *Legionella* prevention programs); pressure relationships and air exchange rates; and the use of high efficiency particulate air filters, with a side discussion of sick building syndrome.

Chapter 6, "Construction and Renovation," focuses on IC issues related to construction and renovation of health care facilities, including IC risk assessment, health care worker education, air quality during construction, risk reduction design elements, and the interdisciplinary approach to minimizing risk in all stages of building projects. The importance of the chapter is significant. During the past six years, the hospital industry has spent more than $100 billion in inflation-adjusted dollars on new facilities, a 47% increase from the previous six years, according to the U.S. Census Bureau.

Chapter 7, "Emergency Management," discusses specifics surrounding surge capacity and the process of decontaminating persons who have been exposed to infectious agents accidentally or through acts of bioterrorism. The pros and cons of indoor and outdoor decontamination are weighed, and solutions for staff training are provided.

Chapter 8, "Performance Measurement and Improvement," focuses on performance improvement in the environmental aspects of IC. It includes strategies for measuring for improvements in the EC and IC so that health care organizations can make and sustain progress, no matter the setting.

Throughout the book, the use of policies, procedures, and guidelines are provided to help you organize and benchmark IC efforts with plans that have proven effective elsewhere. Useful resources and Web sites are listed to help you further examine key subjects.

All health care organizations and facilities are responsible for establishing preventive measures and identification methods for, and elimination and mitigation of, IC risks in its own environment. Some risks are the same in all environments; others are particular to the individual facility. Most organizations will find a useful combination of strategies and approaches described in this book, including those developed by professional and regulatory organizations, and strategies devised through long experience by organizations.

IC is a complex and critical matter in all health care settings including ambulatory care, behavioral health care, long term care, and home care. The term *health care organization* is used to recognize and include these organizations, in addition to the hospital setting.

Acknowledgments

Joint Commission Resources thanks reviewers John Fishbeck, Kelly Fugate, Jerry Gervais, Louise Kuhny, Barbara Soule, Susan Slavish, Diane Bell, Catherine Hinckley, and Paul Reis.

References

1. Centers for Disease Control and Prevention: *Estimates of Healthcare-Associated Infections.* http://www.cdc.gov/ncidod/dhqp/hai.html (accessed Jan. 13, 2009).

2. World Health Organization: *Evidence for Hand Hygiene Guidelines.* http://www.who.int/gpsc/tools/faqs/evidence_hand_hygiene/en (accessed Jan. 13, 2009).

3. Centers for Medicare & Medicaid Services. *Hospital-Acquired Conditions: Present on Admission Indicator.* http://www.cms.hhs.gov/HospitalAcqCond/06_Hospital-Acquired_Conditions.asp (accessed Feb. 3, 2009).

Chapter 1

Making the Connection:
Infection Prevention and Control
and Environment of Care Issues

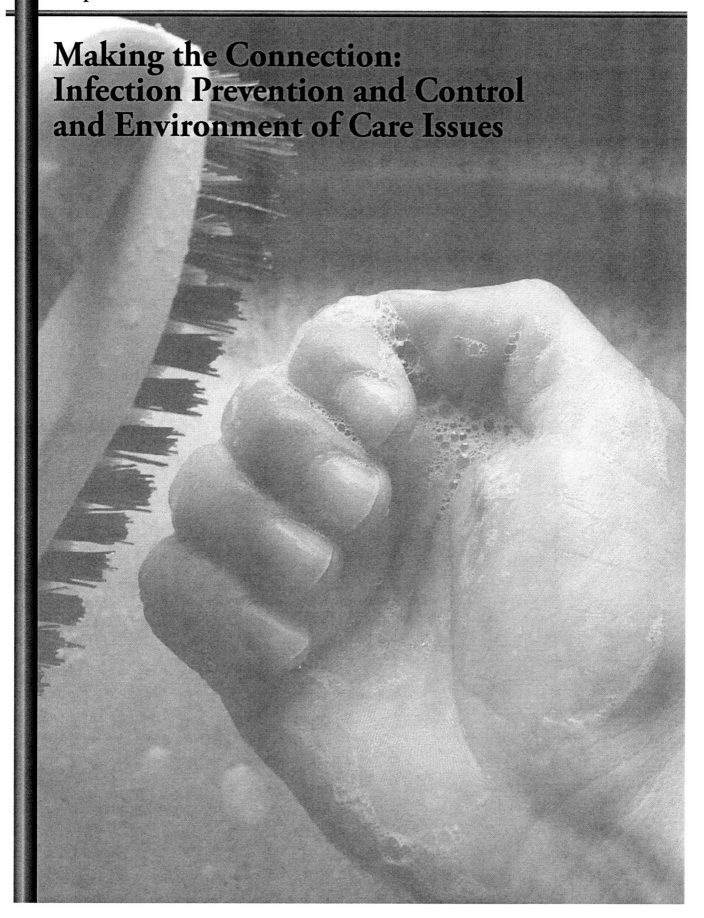

Making the Connection: Infection Prevention and Control and Environment of Care Issues

Patients getting sick or sicker while in a health care setting may be ironic, but it is not new. Some 270 patients die every day from health care–associated infections (HAIs), perhaps a third of them preventable, in addition to the human cost: Treating 2 million patients who acquire HAIs every year costs nearly $5 billion annually.[1] The Joint Commission has made protecting patients from HAIs a top priority through its standards and other initiatives. This chapter introduces the following:

- The Joint Commission's requirements for infection prevention and control (IC)
- Its IC-related environment of care (EC) standards
- Its National Patient Safety Goals related to IC and EC
- The role of the infection preventionist and EC counterpart
- The connection between the IC and EC standards
- The role of the *Life Safety Code*[1] (LSC) specialist
- The role of the EC tour and the IC/EC tracer

Joint Commission Infection Prevention and Control Standards

An effective IC program requires the support and involvement of organization leadership, emphasizes organizationwide communication and collaboration, and includes everyone involved in the organization's daily operations—including care providers and all non-clinical staff. An IC program must meet the needs of the organization's location, services, and population served. The Joint Commission's Infection Prevention and Control standards are designed to help health care organizations develop and maintain effective IC programs regardless of organization size and situation. The standards also call for ongoing risk assessment and monitoring that feature performance measures. In short, the IC standards address planning, implementation, and evaluation steps for creating and maintaining an effective IC program (*see* Sidebar 1-1, page 4, for an overview of the IC standards).

Planning

Planning begins when leadership assigns one person or a team of people (including employees, contractors, and/or consultants) to develop the program. This individual gathers key team members with expertise in IC and facilities management to perform a risk assessment. An IC team will prioritize results of the organization's infection risk assessment, set goals for reducing the risks, and plan focused activities/action plans based on professional guidelines and scientific practices.

More specifically, the planning standards require that the organization have an IC plan developed using evidence-based national guidelines and/or expert consensus, including a written description of activities that include surveillance and the process for evaluating the plan. The organization provides access to information needed to support the IC plan, and identifies, prioritizes, documents, and at least annually reviews the organization's risk for acquiring and transmitting infections based on the following:

- Geographic location
- Population served
- Care, treatment, and services it provides
- Analysis of surveillance activities and other IC data

The written IC goals include the following:

- Addressing the organization's prioritized risks
- Limiting unprotected exposure of patients, visitors, and staff to pathogens
- Limiting the transmission of infections associated with procedures
- Limiting the transmission of infections associated with the use of medical equipment
- Improving compliance with hand hygiene guidelines

[1]*Life Safety Code*® is a registered trademark of the National Fire Protection Association, Quincy, MA.

The IC plan should integrate all of the organization's components and functions, describing the process for investigating outbreaks of infectious disease, and the methods for communicating responsibilities and reporting data to external organizations. The organization should be prepared to respond to an infectious outbreak or influx of infectious patients, and should obtain current information regarding new and emergent infections.

Implementation

To implement the IC plan, the IC team should take practical actions, emphasizing collaboration and communication among departments and staff, and clearly defining roles. When implementing the program, standard- and transmission-based precautions should be used, and IC information should be made available to all staff as well as patients and their families.

Implementation also requires that the organization investigate outbreaks of infectious disease, minimize the risk of infection when storing and disposing of infectious waste, and implement methods to communicate responsibilities for preventing and controlling infection to staff, patients, and their families.

The organization should determine risk of infections associated with use, storage, and disposal of medical equipment, devices, and supplies, and work to prevent the transmission of infectious disease among patients, licensed independent practitioners, and staff by screening for exposure and/or immunity to infectious disease. When staff or patients have or are suspected of having an infectious disease that puts others at risk, the organization should provide or refer them for assessment, testing, immunization, treatment, or counseling.

In addition, the organization offers vaccination against influenza to licensed independent practitioners and staff by establishing an annual influenza vaccination program and educates staff about influenza and vaccinations. The organization should also annually evaluate vaccination rates and the reasons given by staff declining influenza vaccination, and take steps to increase influenza vaccination rates.

Sidebar 1-1: Infection Prevention and Control-Related Standards

The following is a summary of The Joint Commission's IC standards. It is important to consult your program's comprehensive accreditation manual for specific standards and requirements regarding your specific health care setting.

- Identify individuals or positions within the organization that will have the authority to take the appropriate steps in prevention or control of transmission of infectious agents.

- This individual should have clinical authority over the IC program.

- He or she consults with someone who has expertise in IC in order to make informed decisions.

- The number of individuals and skill mix for IC are determined by the goals and objectives of IC activities.

- Adequate resources are allocated to IC.

- Leaders have identified risks for the acquisition and transmission of infectious agents. This is an ongoing activity.

- Risks associated with development of a health care–associated infection should be identified and minimized.

- The IC plan should illustrate the following components:
  - Evidence-based national guidelines
  - Written descriptions of activities
  - Written descriptions of how processes are evaluated
  - Written processes for investigating outbreaks of infectious diseases
  - Integration of all applicable organizational components and functions

- Communication methods are established to report IC issues to licensed independent practitioners, staff, visitors, patients, and families. Methods of how infection surveillance and control information are reported to external organizations are established.

- Implement strategies to prevent the transmission of infectious diseases in the organization's population, with licensed independent practitioners, and with staff.

- The organization is prepared to respond to a higher quantity of a potentially infectious population.

- Reduce the risk of infections associated with medical equipment, devices, and supplies.

- Offer and encourage immunization against influenza to staff and licensed independent practitioners.

- Evaluate the effectiveness of the IC plan.

Evaluation

Continual improvement and evaluation are crucial components of an effective IC program. The IC team should continuously review the organization's goals, activities, and outcomes. Such assessments should be followed up with realistic and effective improvement activities.

The IC standards require that organizations evaluate the effectiveness of their IC plan on an annual basis and whenever risks significantly change. The evaluation is to include a review of the IC prioritized risks, goals, and implementation of activities. Findings from the evaluation are communicated at least annually to the individuals or interdisciplinary group that manage the patient safety program. The organization uses these findings when revising the IC plan.

Joint Commission Environment of Care Standards

A health care organization's environment of care encompasses the physical environment in which patient care, treatment, and services take place. This physical environment includes the building or space and its arrangement and features; the equipment used to operate the building and support patient care; and the activities involved in maintaining a safe and functional environment for patients, visitors, and staff. The "Environment of Care" (EC) chapter helps organizations achieve a safe environment of care, minimizing risk and ensuring a functional space.

The EC standards include requirements for planning, implementing, evaluating improvements, and minimizing risk in the following areas:

- Safety and security
- Use of hazardous materials and waste
- Fire safety
- Use of medical equipment
- Inspection and testing of utilities
- Renovation, demolition, and/or construction projects

The standards require that an individual or group of individuals manage environmental risks and intervene when situations threaten people or property. Several of the EC standards address IC-related issues (*see* Sidebar 1-2, right). The following sections take a further look at the EC standards that relate to IC.

Hazardous Chemicals and Waste

The organization must manage and minimize risks related to selecting, handling, storing, transporting, using, and disposing

---

Sidebar 1-2: Environment of Care Standards Addressing Infection Prevention and Control

The following is a summary of The Joint Commission's EC standards regarding IC. It is important to consult your program's comprehensive accreditation manual for specific standards and requirements regarding your specific health care setting.

- The organization manages risks related to hazardous materials and waste.
- The organization manages medical equipment risks.
- The organization inspects, tests, and maintains medical equipment.
- The organization manages risks associated with its utility systems.
- The organization has a reliable emergency electrical power source.
- The organization inspects, tests, and maintains utility systems.
- The organization inspects, tests, and maintains emergency power systems.
- The organization inspects, tests, and maintains medical gas and vacuum systems.
- The organization establishes and maintains a safe, functional environment.
- The organization manages its environment during demolition, renovation, or new construction to reduce risk to those in the organization.

---

of hazardous chemicals, radioactive materials, hazardous energy sources, hazardous medications, and/or hazardous gases and vapors. To do this, an organization is required to create and maintain a written current inventory of all the hazardous materials and waste it uses, stores, transports, or generates. Written procedures regarding hazardous material and waste spills or exposures should be implemented, including those that relate to the use of precautions and personal protective equipment. In addition, the organization has the permits, licenses, manifests, and material safety data sheets required by law and regulation.

Medical Equipment Use and Risk

The EC standards require organizations to manage medical equipment risks by maintaining either a written inventory of *all* medical equipment or a written inventory of *selected* equipment categorized by physical risk associated with the equipment's use and incident history. Organizations with a limited number of pieces of medical equipment, such as an ambulatory clinic, may elect to keep all possible equipment in the program regardless of risk. But many organizations have a proliferation of equipment, and keeping a detailed record of all possible pieces on the inventory would result in a virtually unmanageable program.

In addition to maintaining an inventory, the organization should evaluate new equipment before initial use, and identify the activities for maintaining, inspecting, and testing all medical equipment, including frequencies for inspecting, testing, and maintaining medical equipment based on criteria such as manufacturers' recommendations, risk levels, or current organization experience. The organization must also monitor and report all incidents in which medical equipment is suspected in or attributed to the death, serious injury, or serious illness of any individual as required by the Safe Medical Devices Act of 1990, and develop written procedures to follow when medical equipment fails, including using emergency clinical interventions and backup equipment.

The organization must also inspect, test, and maintain all medical equipment, including sterilizers and water used in hemodialysis. All inspections, tests, and maintenance must be documented.

Utility Systems

The organization must manage risks associated with its utility systems and design, and install systems that meet patient care and operational needs. As with medical equipment, organizations must maintain a written inventory of *all* operating components of their utility systems or *selected* critical components based on risks for infection, occupant needs, and systems critical to patient care. The organization must evaluate new types of utility components and identify activities for all operating components of utility systems including intervals for inspection, testing, and maintenance based on criteria such as manufacturer's recommendations, risk levels, or organization experience. The organization must minimize pathogenic biological agents in cooling towers and water systems and in areas designed to control airborne contaminants, ensuring the ventilation system provides appropriate pressure relationships, air-exchange rates, and filtration efficiencies. In addition, the organization must map distribution of its utility systems and label utility system controls to facilitate partial or complete emergency shut downs, and develop written procedures for responding to

system disruptions, including shutting off the malfunctioning system and notifying staff in affected areas. Procedures must address communicating the need for emergency clinical interventions during utility systems disruptions and how to obtain emergency repair services.

Emergency Power Sources

The organization must maintain a reliable emergency electrical power source for alarm systems; exit route and exit sign illumination; emergency communication systems; elevators; and equipment that could cause patient harm when it fails, including life support systems, blood, bone, and tissue storage systems, medical air compressors, and medical and surgical vacuum systems. Also, areas in which loss of power could result in patient harm, including operating rooms, recovery rooms, obstetrical delivery rooms, nurseries, and urgent care areas must have a reliable emergency electrical power source.

The organization must also inspect, test, and maintain emergency power systems, medical gas and vacuum systems, and new utility systems and components on the inventory before initial use. In addition, the organization must test and maintain life support utility system components, IC utility system components, and non-life support utility system components, and document these activities.

Safe and Functional Environment

The organization must establish and maintain a safe, functional environment. Interior spaces must meet needs of the patient population and be safe and suitable to the care, treatment, and services provided. Lighting, ventilation, temperature, and humidity levels must be maintained.

Demolition, Renovation and/or Construction

The organization must manage its environment during demolition, renovation, or new construction to reduce risk to those in the organization. When planning for a new, altered, or renovated space, organizations should consult state rules and regulations, the *Guidelines for Design and Construction of Hospitals and Health Care Facilities, 2001 edition,* and other current construction guidelines. Preconstruction risk assessment for air quality and utility requirements, as well as infection risks, noise, vibration, and other hazards that affect care, treatment, and services must be conducted before renovation or construction projects begin, and the organization must take action based on its assessment to minimize risk during any such projects.

National Patient Safety Goal 7 and Infection Prevention and Control

The Joint Commission's commitment to IC does not begin or end with the standards. Its accreditation process is also complemented by the National Patient Safety Goals. Specifically, National Patient Safety Goal 7 requires organizations to reduce the risk of health care–associated infections, and organizations must meet the applicable requirements of this IC-related goal. (*see* Sidebar 1-3, right).

National Patient Safety Goal 7 requires that health care organizations comply with current World Health Organization or Centers for Disease Control and Prevention hand hygiene guidelines to reduce the transmission of infectious agents by staff to patients, thereby decreasing the incidence of health care–associated infections. Although there are many ways to approach hand hygiene compliance efforts, one EC-related approach involves technology and design features developed to overcome staff cognitive or behavioral resistance to hand hygiene compliance. Such technology and design features may include the following:

- Recorded reminders to wash hands before entering or leaving a patient room
- A flashing light reminder to wash hands when entering or leaving a patient room
- Installing sinks directly in the caregiver's work path
- Installing alcohol-based hand rub dispensers just inside and outside patient rooms, treatment rooms, suites, and other appropriate locations

National Patient Safety Goal 7 requires that health care organizations manage as sentinel events all identified cases of unanticipated death or major permanent loss of function associated with an HAI. A root cause analysis (RCA) is required in response to a patient acquiring the infection. An RCA can help determine the relationship between a patient's care process and an HAI by reviewing the patient experience and determining when or how an HAI was acquired, and whether the death or loss of function is related to the HAI. Analyzing features of the EC, such as design, overall safety, handling of hazardous materials, and medical equipment, will be essential to any such RCA.

Goal 7 also requires implementation of evidence-based practices to prevent multiple drug-resistant organisms (MDRO) infections in organizations. Risks and patient populations vary among health care organizations, so prevention and control strategies must be tailored to the specific needs of each organization based on the organization's risk assessment. That said, some common best practices to prevent MDRO infections include the following:

- Conducting periodic risk assessments for MDRO acquisition and transmission. Risk assessments should involve evaluating both the EC and clinical practice.
- Implementing policies and practices aimed at reducing MDRO risk, meeting regulatory requirements, and aligning with evidence-based standards.
- Implementing a surveillance program.
- Providing surveillance data to key stakeholders.
- Developing a laboratory-based alert system for patients with MDROs (if risk assessment indicates a need).
- Developing an alert system for identifying readmitted or transferred MDRO-positive patients (if risk assessment indicates a need).
- Educating staff about MDROs in a manner consistent with staff's organizational roles.
- Educating patients and families as needed. It is essential that EC issues be considered when educating patients and staff regarding MDROs.
- Measuring and monitoring MDRO prevention and outcomes.

Sidebar 1-3: IC-Related National Patient Safety Goal 7

The following is a summary of The Joint Commission's National Patient Safety Goal 7. It is important to consult your program's comprehensive accreditation manual for specific National Patient Safety Goals requirements regarding your specific health care setting.

- Reduce the risk of health care–associated infections.

- Comply with current World Health Organization hand hygiene guidelines or Centers for Disease Control and Prevention hand hygiene guidelines.

- Manage as sentinel events all identified cases of unanticipated death or major permanent loss of function related to a health care–associated infection.

- Implement evidence-based practices to prevent health care–associated infections due to multidrug-resistant organisms in acute care organizations.

- Implement best practices or evidence-based guidelines to prevent central line-associated bloodstream infections

- Implement best practices for preventing surgical site infections.

Goal 7 also requires implementation of best practices or evidence-based guidelines to prevent central line-associated bloodstream infections (CLABSI) and surgical site infections (SSI). Consistent with EC and IC standards, this goal requires that staff involved in these processes be educated about HAIs and prevention. In addition, implementing and periodically updating policies and practices that both meet regulatory requirements and are aligned with evidence-based standards will require revisiting IC outcomes and their relationship to the EC. For example, how medical equipment is supplied to the room and whether personal protective equipment is available in patient rooms may affect rates of CLABSI and SSI.

Connection Between Environment of Care and Infection Prevention and Control Requirements

Effective implementation of IC measures and methods requires a multidisciplinary process and team that includes the EC professional. In addition to clinical staff, collaborators typically include representatives from environmental services, safety, housekeeping, equipment maintenance, building maintenance and engineering, and laundry services.

Representatives of these services often meet together either informally or formally on an IC team or task force to discuss IC issues. Such a multidisciplinary body can draw on expertise from many sources as a good way to involve the entire organization in the effort to prevent infections.

Although the EC is much less frequently implicated than direct physical contact or care processes in disease transmission, it is clear that organisms live and survive in patient care environments, sometimes for very long periods. *Staphylococcus aureus* and *Clostridium difficile* are two examples. These organisms may be transferred to patients by the hands of staff or from equipment. Other organisms, such as *Legionella*, can live in the facility's water supply and can cause severe outbreaks of infections. Still others, such as *Aspergillus* species, can be transmitted during construction and can severely affect the health of immunocompromised patients. Environmental strategies and engineering controls can help prevent inadvertent exposures to these pathogens. These strategies include the following[2]:
- Appropriate use of cleaning and disinfectant agents and frequent cleaning of environmental surfaces

- Appropriate maintenance and cleaning of medical equipment
- Adherence to water quality standards for hemodialysis and ventilation standards for specialized care environments (airborne infection isolation rooms, operating rooms)
- Prompt management of water intrusion into the facility, including mold abatement
- Appropriate precautions and barriers during construction and renovation. Chapter 6, "Construction and Renovation," further addresses this topic.

Occupational health statistics on employee exposure to infectious diseases, tests for seroconversions from exposure to tubercle bacilli, rates and types of sharps injuries, and employee exposures to blood and other body fluids can help make EC and IC professionals aware of issues that can be monitored and controlled to increase worker safety. Trending and disseminating such data can validate effective programs and point out where other programs might be improved.

EC workers should collaborate with IC preventionists in addressing potential contamination related to areas such as drains, ice machines, carpeting and flooring, ceiling tiles and the space above them, elevator shafts, receiving, and garbage or medical waste storage areas (also *see* Chapter 3, "Equipment").

EC and IC professionals should be present during all stages of construction and renovation projects—from review of the design and scope of the project through the completion and acceptance of the project by all parties. Although their separate expertise is needed to address air handling needs, protective barriers, and debris removal, they often overlap and enhance each other's contributions. The typical collaborative relationship between EC and IC occurs when the following is needed:
- Handling of hazardous materials and waste
- Creation of contingency plans for interrupted utility services
- Analysis of infectious disease risks with use of biomedical equipment
- Analysis of IC measures during physical plant renovation, alteration, or new construction

The Environment of Care Tour

In order to determine whether an organization's management of safety risks is effective and whether safety policies and procedures are actually practiced and enforced, all health care organizations are required to conduct regular environmental tours. Because the EC plays a major role in preventing infections, an EC tour can help identify IC issues. For example, the EC tour team might discover construction or renovation barriers that are not working correctly, ventilation systems that need maintenance, or isolation rooms in which negative air pressure is not working correctly. Cracked floors, countertops, or furniture, as well as sinks that regularly splash water onto the floor requires attention and are potential sources for germs or bacteria to grow and infect patient rooms, caregivers, and patients.

During an EC tour, all areas of all facilities—ideally including grounds—are visited and evaluated for environmental deficiencies, hazards, and unsafe practices at least once a year. Patient care areas are evaluated every six months. Since many departments, including IC, must tour the facility to gather data, validate current practices, and identify areas for improvement, an EC tour is an excellent opportunity to inspect buildings, grounds, and activities collaboratively. An efficient tour includes as many functions in a single tour as possible and can include assessments of the following areas:

- *Life Safety Code* (National Fire Protection Association [NFPA] 101)
- Environmental services
- IC efforts (such as those related to utilities, equipment, or renovation sites)
- Occupational Safety and Health Administration and workers' compensation issues
- Clinical issues
- Patient safety

Elements of the Environment of Care Tour

The environmental tour should be conducted by a person or persons involved in coordinating EC, written into policy, scheduled carefully, and include both checklists and forms for documenting and resolving discrepancies. The written policy might include frequency of tours and members of the tour team. The makeup of a tour team might look like the following:

- Administration
- Clinical staff

- Safety and facilities management
- Quality or risk management
- Biomedical engineering
- Housekeeping
- IC professional

Not every organization will have different people in these various roles, but having each role represented, where appropriate, is advisable.

The environmental tour is a good opportunity for team members to question staff members about their roles in EC management. Depending on staff response, the environmental tour team can identify priority areas for future education programs. The tour policy should describe:

- Steps to be followed
- Data to be collected, analyzed, and used
- Follow-up process for identified problem areas
- Mechanism for reporting tour results to EC coordinators and organizationwide
- Use of re-inspection/correction reports to verify improvement

In addition, creating a tour schedule or calendar that explicitly covers all areas of the facility will ensure that no area is left unvisited. Indeed, leaving the tours to chance virtually assures that they will be incomplete. Likewise, the environmental tour team should develop checklists to ensure that important areas are thoroughly covered on each tour (*see* Figure 1-1, on page 11 for a sample checklist of IC issues). Discrepancy forms for documenting inconsistencies or problem areas will enable the environmental tour team to inform staff who need to correct the problem(s) and track improvements. These forms can serve as review documents to make sure corrections have been made.

Joint Commission Tracer

The Joint Commission uses tracer methodology to analyze a health care organization's system of providing care, treatment, and services using actual patients as the framework for assessing standards compliance. Within this methodology, surveyors follow the experience of care for a number of individuals through the organization's entire health care process. This allows the surveyor(s) to identify performance issues in one or more steps of the process, or in the interfaces between steps.

Tracers involve assessment, discussion, and education about many areas of organization performance, including IC and EC. There are many ways surveyors assess IC and EC within tracers. For example, the surveyor can provide guidance to an organization and its staff by evaluating the systems and performance for managing risk in the EC, life safety, and emergency care. Such evaluation will assist the organization with the following:

- Identifying areas of concern/risk in the EC/IC
- Identifying organizational strengths in preventing/ mitigating risk in the EC/IC
- Assessing actual compliance with EC/IC standards
- Determining actions necessary for addressing areas of concern

During a tracer, the surveyor may identify a vulnerable area in the organization's EC or IC and trace the risk through the organization's management processes. Health care organizations can expect the surveyor to pose any number of questions during a tracer that may relate to the EC and IC. For example, if an organization's vulnerable area involves the EC issue of maintaining ventilation systems, the potential transmission of respiratory infections is obviously quite high. Similarly, EC issues such as maintaining clean water sources and storage of hazardous materials/medical equipment are also directly linked to the organization's IC efforts.

Within tracer activities, the organization will discuss with the surveyor(s) how the following EC functional areas are addressed within the organization:

- General safety and security
- Hazardous materials and waste
- Fire safety
- Medical/laboratory equipment
- Utilities
- Other environmental considerations

In addition, the surveyor(s) will review the organization's management processes for the following:

- Identify risks in the EC/IC
- Communicating staff roles and responsibilities
- Implementing procedures and controls for minimizing risk
- Determining organizational response for an EC failure/ incident
- Monitoring EC/IC performance
- Improving EC/IC performance

Depending on the organization, surveyors may evaluate IC issues as part of an IC-specific tracer, in part to determine the strengths and vulnerabilities of the organization's IC plan. Within this tracer, questions may directly relate to the EC as well as the IC and may include the following:

- Does the organization have plans in place to reduce the risk of infections associated with medical equipment, devices, and supplies?
- How would the organization handle infection risks if utilities were not available—for example, how would hand hygiene be performed without a water source?
- How does the organization work to prevent the transmission of infectious diseases, including those caused by waterborne and airborne pathogens?

Another way surveyors can identify EC and IC issues during the onsite survey is through the *Life Safety Code* assessment. The *Life Safety Code* is the NFPA standards that specify construction and operational conditions to minimize fire hazards and provide a system of safety in case of fire. The Joint Commission requires certain health care settings—including hospitals and long term care organizations—to comply with the *Life Safety Code*. One purpose of the LSC assessment is to gauge compliance with the LSC requirements that may pose a threat to the patient, staff, and visitors in the EC.

LSC-related issues associated with the EC and IC requirements include the following:

- Hazardous areas, such as soiled linen rooms, trash collection rooms, oxygen storage rooms, and kitchens
- Condition of all emergency power systems and equipment
- Verification that there is a reliable emergency power system when normal power supply is interrupted
- Medical gas and vacuum components

For hospitals and critical access hospitals, the *Life Safety Code* assessment is conducted by the LSC specialist. This individual is a member of the survey team and has a professional background as a facility engineer, safety manager, or other EC professional. Because of this background, he or she is able to provide a detailed focus on life safety conditions in a hospital.

It is the job of the LSC specialist to investigate and communicate all issues related to the LSC to the organization. Specifically, the LSC specialist is responsible for evaluating

Figure 1-1: Sample Infection Prevention and Control Monitor Checklist

This figure provides a sample checklist of some EC issues from which organizations can begin to design their own risk-specific checklist.

Unit _____

Monitor _____

Date _____

Item	Yes	No	N/A
Clean linens are stored in covered carts			
Hand wash areas are equipped with paper towels, trash receptacles, and appropriate soap.			
Hand rub gel dispensers are filled and placed in and near patient care areas and public access areas			
Sharps receptacle containers are secured and no more than three-quarters full			
Only disinfectants approved for health care are present, and they are used according to the manufacturer's directions			
High-level disinfection/sterilization monitoring logs are up-to-date			
Face shields/goggles/personal protective equipment are available and used during procedures and cleaning			
Signs are posted indicating restricted eating or drinking where and when care is delivered			
Hand wash areas are equipped with paper towels, trash receptacles, and appropriate soap			
No patient care supplies are stored on the floor or under sinks			
Negative pressure rooms are available for isolation, as needed			
In areas under construction, infection prevention and control and risk reduction interventions are in place			

Comments _____

_____

EC and LSC requirements, identifying compliance issues and opportunities for improvement, discussing any remedial action that may be required, and consulting with organizations to address compliance in the long term. The LSC specialist assesses compliance through interviews, document review, and the LSC tour, in which he or she tours the building and grounds assessing compliance with LSC-related standards. A staff member should be prepared to answer any LSC questions, even if he/she is not an EC professional. Compliance with the LSC—as with IC and EC standard requirements—requires that leadership and staff be familiar with the relationship between EC and the risk of infection or harm; continually evaluate and monitor best practices and evidence-based guidelines for meeting regulatory requirements; and periodically assess risk, areas of vulnerability, and opportunities for improvement.

Role of the Environment of Care Professional and Infection Preventionist

An organization's EC professional and infection preventionist play a central role in maintaining a safe health care environment that complies with EC and IC standards and requirements. These specialized professionals can help in prevention efforts by connecting the science of IC and EC to the people and areas most deeply affected. An infection preventionist will be in close communication with EC professionals. An infection preventionist will be a close partner to EC professionals to ensure space and building safety; to evaluate, purchase, and maintain ventilation systems and water systems; and to ensure proper handling, storage, and disposal of hazardous wastes and resources used by the organization. EC professionals and infection preventionists must have a keen understanding of how the EC—construction and renovation projects, ventilation, building space, utilities and use, storage, and disposal of hazardous materials and waste, energy sources, and so on—can be manipulated, planned, and/or designed to minimize risk of infection to everyone who enters and plays a role in the environment. Infection preventionists and EC professionals are jointly involved in ensuring a clean, safe building that minimizes IC and EC risks.

EC professionals and infection preventionists are faced with numerous demands, and yet minimizing, and where possible eliminating, HAIs is an important aspect of both the IC and EC professionals' role. HAIs on which IC and EC professionals should focus include central line-associated bloodstream infection (CLABSI), ventilator-associated pneumonia, catheter-associated urinary tract infection, surgical site infection, infection caused by MDROs, such as methicillin-resistant *Staphylococcus aureus* and *Clostridium difficile*, and other transmittable infections (*see* Sidebar 1-4, page 13, for definitions of infections). To reduce and eliminate HAIs, IC and EC professionals must manage environmental practices and factors, including facility cleanliness, good ventilation, water free from serious pathogens, and adherence to policies and regulations for IC-related construction and renovation projects. Such management also includes ongoing surveillance of environmental issues and working to ensure that infection outbreaks related to the environment are minimized or eliminated in order to diminish their effect on patient outcomes and an organization's bottom line.[3]

Although IC and EC professionals play a critical role in preventing and eliminating HAIs, the responsibility for this effort is not solely bared by these professionals. All individuals who enter a health care organization—staff, patients, visitors, licensed independent practitioners, and others—must be involved in preventing the spread of infection and embrace their role in IC efforts. Organizations can support participation in IC interventions by eliminating the barriers to participation and making it easier to engage in best practices. In other words, organizations can address the "human factors" involved in IC activities—the behaviors, abilities, limitations, and environmental distractions that impact an individual's ability to participate effectively in activities. Chapter 2 begins the discussion of the relationship between IC efforts and human factors, specifically focusing on hand hygiene and education and training strategies.

Sidebar 1-4: Environment of Care and Common Health Care–Associated Infections (HAIs)

One goal of an effective IC program is to reduce the risk of acquiring and transmitting HAIs. Although there are many HAIs, the following is a brief description of some with which organizations should be familiar:

- **Methicillin-resistant *Staphylococcus aureus* (MRSA)**—*Staphylococcus aureus*, also known as "Staph," is a very common organism that many people have on their skin or in their noses. When staph become resistant to methicillin (a common antibiotic), this germ can cause serious infections of the skin, blood, lungs, or wounds. MRSA infections are harder to treat because fewer antibiotics are effective once the *Staphylococci* become resistant.

- ***Clostridium difficile* infection**—*Clostridium difficile*, also known as *C. diff*, is a type of bacteria that causes diarrhea and, in some cases, more serious intestinal infections. *C. diff* can increases hospital stays as well as costs, morbidity, and mortality in adult patients, and has been linked with environmental transmission. *C. diff* is found in feces. Any surface, device, or material that becomes contaminated with feces, such as toilet seats, bathing tubs, and electronic rectal thermometers, may serve as a reservoir for *C. diff* spores.

- **Central line-associated bloodstream infection (CLABSI)**—Patients, particularly those requiring intensive care, often need central lines (also called central venous catheters) for fluids or medications. A CLABSI occurs when microorganisms travel through or around the catheter and enter the blood. This can lead to serious illness or mortality and longer hospitalization.

- **Ventilator-associated pneumonia (VAP)**—VAP occurs in patients who require a machine to help them breathe. An estimated 25% of patients on ventilator support will develop VAP. The position of the bed, poor oral care, and length of time on the ventilator has all been associated with increased incidence of VAP.

- **Catheter-associated urinary tract infection (CAUTI)**—Urinary catheters are used for patients unable to urinate on their own. Urinary tract infection is the most common HAI, with about 80% of urinary tract infections acquired in the hospital attributable to long-term use of urinary catheters.

- **Surgical site infection (SSI)**—SSI occurs in 2% to 5% of patients undergoing inpatient surgery in the United States, with an estimated 500,000 occurring annually. Overall, SSIs are associated with about $7 billion to $10 billion annually in health care expenditures in the United States.[4] Poor hand hygiene, incomplete surgical preparation, and inconsistent use of presurgical antibiotics can increase the likelihood of SSI.

There are many environmental strategies and engineering controls that can help prevent inadvertent exposure to pathogens, such as the ones listed above. These environmental strategies include, but are not limited to, the following:

- Appropriate use of cleaners and disinfectants

- Maintenance of medical equipment

- Appropriate and consistent hand hygiene

- Adherence to water quality and ventilation standards

- Prompt management of water intrusion

References

1. Centers for Disease Control and Prevention: *Estimates of Health Care-Acquired Infections.* http://www.cdc.gov/ncidod/dhqp/hai.html (accessed Jun. 10, 2009).

2. Sehulster, L. Chinn R.Y.W.: Guidelines for environmental infection control in health-care facilities: Recommendations of CDC and Healthcare Infection Control Practices Advisory Committee (HICPAC). *MMWR Recommendations and Reports*, 52 (RR10), Jun. 6, 2003. http://www.cdc.gov/ncidod/dhqp/gl_environinfection.html (accessed Jun. 12, 2009).

3. Pittet D., Donaldson L.: Challenging the world: Patient safety and health care-associated infection. *Int J Qual Health Care* 18(1):4-8, 2006.

4. Society for Healthcare Epidemiology of America, Infectious Diseases Society of America, American Hospital Association, Association for Professionals in Infection Control and Epidemiology, The Joint Commission: Nation's Top Healthcare Organizations Announce Strategies to Prevent Deadly Healthcare-Associated Infections. Oct. 8, 2008. http://www.apic.org/AM/Template.cfm/Section=Featured_News_and_Events&CONTENTID=11957&TEMPMLATE=/CM/ContentDisplay.cfm (accessed Jun. 12, 2009).

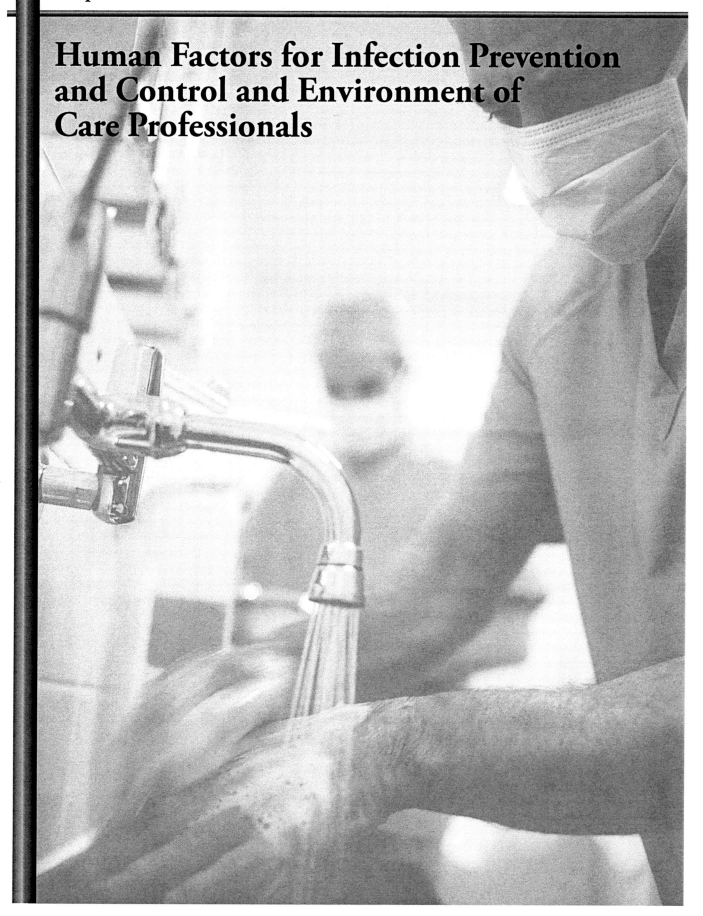

Chapter 2

Human Factors for Infection Prevention and Control and Environment of Care Professionals

Human Factors for Infection Prevention and Control and Environment of Care Professionals

Infection prevention and control (IC) has benefited from innovation in so many ways—from waterless hand hygiene products and safety needles and disposal systems to new germicides. But without trained, motivated, professional workers, these developments are useless. In the same manner, infection preventionists are unable to keep health care–associated infections (HAIs) at bay without the cooperation of all employees in an organization, including clinical and nonclinical staff. Like other aspects of safety, IC is everybody's responsibility, including the patient (*see* Sidebar 2-1, page 18).

All employees must consistently adhere to organization policies and procedures, be aware of potential exposures, and know how to respond if they experience or witness a breach of protocol in protecting themselves, patients, and visitors. As this chapter stresses, staff must be prepared to work together as team members when the occasion demands, to minimize contamination in an emergency, to remind each other to wash their hands and use personal protective equipment (PPE), and to share expertise on IC committees and task forces. With this in mind, the pages ahead focus on IC and environment of care (EC) collaboration, the importance of hand hygiene, and the methods of IC staff training and education.

The Infection Prevention and Control and Environment of Care Affiliation

As touched on in the preceding chapters, one of the most fruitful collaborations in the context of IC is that of the infection preventionists and EC professionals. Each group forms a natural partnership in IC hazard assessment, product selection, data collection, facility monitoring, and emergency management—including decontamination activities. Ideally, the infection preventionist and EC professional will be trained together in IC principles and practices where areas of responsibility overlap and to maintain open communication channels between the disciplines.

Collaboration of all relevant components/functions in the organizationwide IC program is vital to the successful gathering and interpretation of data, design of interventions, and effective implementation of interventions in The Joint Commission's IC standards. With leaders and staff in central supply and sterilization services, housekeeping, building maintenance and engineering, and other departments as engaged participants in IC, organizations are better prepared to improve patient safety and care.

Collaborative Relationship

Collaboration as a daily, routine matter is what makes it possible for different disciplines to work together smoothly during emergencies, capitalizing on the understanding built up over time. This is why cross-populating IC and EC committees and having members conduct joint IC/EC rounds makes great sense. It ensures that organizations develop ventilation policies, for example, with the benefit of both perspectives. Committee representatives can bring back to their own groups news about infection transmission issues and recommendations for improvement and report back on progress that has been made.

Collaboration is equally important with all personnel. For example, housekeeping staff who understand the importance of thoroughly cleaning the patient's environment to prevent transmission of potentially pathogenic organisms from inanimate surfaces to patients are more likely to perform their housekeeping duties conscientiously and therefore to feel good about helping to prevent infections and provide safer patient care.

Another step is to have the infection preventionists come to environmental services (ES) staff meetings and provide training on pathogenic microorganism control

Sidebar 2-1: The Role of the Patient

One person that otherwise-vigilant organizations forget to enlist in the infection prevention and control (IC) program is the patient, who can unwittingly undo much of the effort expended by staff unless he or she is educated in the basics of IC. The Joint Commission, together with the Centers for Medicare & Medicaid Services, launched the Speak Up™ Campaign to urge patients to take a role in preventing health care errors by becoming active, involved, and informed participants on the health care team. The program features brochures, posters, and buttons on various patient safety topics including "Five Things You Can Do to Prevent Infection."

The five easy things patients and health care providers can do include:

1. Clean your hands.
2. Make sure health care providers clean their hands or wear gloves.
3. Cover your mouth and nose when you cough or sneeze.
4. If you are sick, avoid close contact with others.
5. Get shots to avoid disease and fight the spread of infection.

In addition, The Joint Commission released "Measuring Hand Hygiene Adherence: Overcoming the Challenges" to help health care organizations target their efforts in measuring hand hygiene performance. The aim of the monograph is to broaden understanding of the issues and provide practical solutions for strengthening measurement and improvement activities.

The monograph is the result of collaboration with infection control leadership organizations in the United States and abroad. In addition to The Joint Commission, the participating organizations include:

- Association for Professionals in Infection Control and Epidemiology, Inc.
- The Centers for Disease Control and Prevention
- The Institute for Healthcare Improvement
- The National Foundation for Infectious Diseases
- The Society for Healthcare Epidemiology of America
- The World Health Organization

The monograph is available at http://www.jointcommission.org/NR/rdonlyres/68B9CB2F-789F-49DB-9E3F-2FB387666BCC/0/hh_monograph.pdf.

The Speak Up materials are available at http://www.jointcommission.org/PatientSafety/SpeakUp and can be downloaded free of charge.

measures. For example, forming a methicillin-resistant *Staphylococcus aureus* (MRSA) risk-reduction task force that includes physicians, nurses, respiratory therapy, infection preventionists, and ES staff could help delegate, monitor, and report usage rates of hand hygiene compliance. In addition to providing valuable information to staff, this type of feedback is consistent with National Patient Safety Goal[1] and the Centers for Disease Control and Prevention (CDC)'s recommendation to monitor hand hygiene compliance.

Hand Hygiene

One basic strategy at the heart of every IC program in every health care setting is to use observation, intuition, and data when monitoring hand washing. Despite more than a century and a half of growing knowledge about the nature and transmission of infections, health care organizations today are wrestling with the same basic challenge (*see* Case Study 2-1, page 31). Although studies show it to be a proven effective practice, hand hygiene compliance among health care workers is poor, with the World Health Organization (WHO) reporting an average compliance rate of 40% (*see* the WHO guidelines on pages 24–26). As the number one defense against health care–acquired conditions, it has been estimated that hand washing alone could prevent 20,000 patient deaths per year.[1] Sidebar 2-2 on page 19 explains the sequence of events associated with the transmittal of pathogens by the hands of health care workers.

Updated in 2008 and based on the recommendations of the Healthcare Infection Control Practices Advisory Committee (HICPAC) and the HICPAC/Society for Healthcare Epidemiology of America/Association for Professionals in Infection Control and Epidemiology (APIC)/Infectious Diseases Society of America Hand Hygiene Task Force, CDC hand hygiene guidelines are outlined in Figure 2-1 (page 20).

The WHO's 2008 *Guidelines on Hand Hygiene in Health Care* advanced draft represents a consensus of international experts and up-to-date technical information on hand hygiene improvements within the health care context across the world. The guidelines are being pilot tested, and it is likely that changes will be made to some of the technical content of the chapters in light of pilot test results. An advanced draft of the guidelines can be downloaded at http://www.who.int/patientsafety/information_centre/guidelines_hhad/en/.

The Handwashing Leadership Forum focuses on reducing the risks of foodborne illness in and outside of health care. But its advice on hand washing behavior is equally sound in constructing a broader IC educational program for infection preventionist and EC professionals. Its recommendations are listed in Sidebar 2-3 on page 23.

Time Issues

The CDC guidelines actively promote the most dramatic development in hand hygiene in recent decades by the introduction of alcohol-based hand rubs to everyday use in the health care setting in the United States. Such hand rubs are considered equivalent in effectiveness to soap and water when hands are not visibly soiled, and offer greater convenience, faster action, and less skin irritation.

The problem with soap and water is not just the need for plumbing, sinks, soap dispensers, and some means of drying hands; it is also the time required to do the job right. In its guidelines, the CDC recommends vigorous rubbing for at least 15 seconds. Observational studies, however, have shown that the average duration of hand-washing episodes in hospitals is less than 15 seconds—indeed, as low as 6.6 seconds—during which time personnel often fail to cover all surfaces of their hands and fingers.[2]

Another problematic aspect of time has to do with feedback. "The gap in time between not performing hand hygiene to the time when the patient gets an infection is days or longer, so staff do not really see the link," explains Elaine Larson, R.N., Ph.D., C.I.C., from the Columbia University School of Nursing. "That's part of the problem; they don't get immediate feedback." This can be especially true of staff in high-risk, high-volume areas of an organization, such as an emergency department or intensive care unit. According to Larson, there is reverse correlation between how sick the patients on a unit are, or how busy the unit is, and how frequently caregivers wash their hands. The high-risk areas where hand hygiene is the most important are the areas where it might be most neglected.

Barriers to Hygiene Practice

In addition to time, the CDC identified the following barriers to adherence with hand hygiene practice recommendations:
- Skin irritation caused by hand hygiene agents
- Inaccessible hand hygiene supplies
- Perception of interference with staff–patient relationships
- Priority of care, that is, putting patients' needs at a higher

---

Sidebar 2-2: Sequence of Events for Transmittal of Pathogens by Hands

Transmission of health care–associated pathogens from one patient to another via the hands of health care workers requires the following sequence of events:

1. Organisms present on the patient's skin, or that have been shed onto inanimate objects in close proximity to the patient, must be transferred to the hands of the health care worker.

2. Organisms must be capable of surviving for at least several minutes on the hands of staff.

3. Hand washing or hand antisepsis by the health care worker must be inadequate or omitted entirely, or the agent used for hand hygiene must be inappropriate.

4. The contaminated hands of the health care worker must come in direct contact with another patient, or with an inanimate object that will come into direct contact with the patient.

Sources: Centers for Disease Control and Prevention: Guideline for Hand Hygiene in Health-Care Settings: Recommendations of the Healthcare Infection Control Practices Advisory Committee and the HICPAC/SHEA/APIC/IDSA Hand Hygiene Task Force. *MMWR Recomm Rep* 51(RR16), Oct. 25, 2002. http://www.cdc.gov/mmwr/preview/mmwrhtml/rr5116a1.htm (accessed Jan. 9, 2009).

World Alliance on Patient Safety: *WHO Guidelines on Hand Hygiene in Health Care (Advanced Draft), Global Patient Safety Challenge 2005–2006: Clean Care Is Safer Care.* 2007. http://www.who.int/patientsafety/information_centre/Last_April_versionHH_Guidelines%5b3%5d.pdf (accessed Jan. 9, 2009).

---

priority than hand hygiene
- Resistance to wearing gloves
- Forgetfulness
- Lack of knowledge of practice guidelines
- Insufficient time
- High work load and understaffing
- Lack of awareness of the risk of cross-transmission of pathogens

Health care organizations have spent considerable time and money to overcome each of these points. Clearly, education is key—education about the relationship between hand hygiene and HAI rates, about the efficacy and use of hand hygiene and skin care protection products, and about hand hygiene guidelines. But just as clearly, the crux of the issue is neither

Figure 2-1: Centers for Disease Control and Prevention (CDC) Guidelines for Hand Hygiene in Health Care Settings

The following is excerpted from the CDC guidelines. The Joint Commission requires implementation of all recommendations supported by Category I evidence, which include all those not marked with an asterisk (indicating Category II evidence). Organizations are asked to consider implementing all recommendations supported by Category II evidence.[2]

- Indications for hand washing and hand antisepsis
  - When hands are visibly dirty or contaminated with proteinaceous material or are visibly soiled with blood or other body fluids, wash hands with either a non-antimicrobial soap and water or an antimicrobial soap and water.
  - If hands are not visibly soiled, use an alcohol-based hand rub for routinely decontaminating hands in all other clinical situations described below. Alternatively, wash hands with an antimicrobial soap and water in all clinical situations described below.
    - Decontaminate hands:
      □ Before having direct contact with patients
      □ Before donning sterile gloves when inserting a central intravascular catheter
      □ Before inserting indwelling urinary catheters, peripheral vascular catheters, or other invasive devices that do not require a surgical procedure
      □ After contact with a patient's intact skin (for example, when taking a pulse or blood pressure, lifting a patient)
      □ After contact with body fluids or excretions, mucous membranes, nonintact skin, and wound dressings if hands are not visibly soiled
      □ If moving from a contaminated-body site to a clean-body site during patient care
      □ After contact with inanimate objects (including medical equipment) in the immediate vicinity of the patient
      □ After removing gloves
      □ Before eating and after using a restroom, wash hands with a non-antimicrobial soap and water or with an antimicrobial soap and water.
  - Antimicrobial-impregnated wipes (that is, towelettes) may be considered as an alternative to washing hands with non-antimicrobial soap and water.
  - Because they are not as effective as alcohol-based hand rubs or washing hands with an antimicrobial soap and water for reducing bacterial counts on the hands of health care workers, antimicrobial wipes are not a substitute for using an alcohol-based hand rub or antimicrobial soap.
  - Wash hands with non-antimicrobial soap and water or with antimicrobial soap and water if exposure to *Bacillus*

anthracis is suspected or proven. The physical action of washing and rinsing hands under such circumstances is recommended because alcohols, chlorhexidrine, iodophors, and other antiseptic agents have poor activity against spores.
  - No recommendation can be made regarding the routine use of non-alcohol-based hand rubs for hand hygiene in health care settings. This is an unresolved issue.[2]

- Hand hygiene technique
  - When decontaminating hands with an alcohol-based hand rub apply product to palm of one hand and rub hands together, covering all surfaces of hands and fingers until hands are dry. Follow the manufacturer recommendations regarding the volume of product to use.
  - When washing hands with soap and water, wet hands first with water, apply an amount of product recommended by the manufacturer to hands, and rub hands together vigorously for at least 15 seconds, covering all surfaces of the hands and fingers. Rinse hands with water and dry thoroughly with a disposable towel. Use towel to turn off the faucet. Avoid using hot water because repeated exposure to hot water may increase the risk of dermatitis.
  - Liquid, bar, leaflet, or powdered forms of plain soap are acceptable when washing hands with a non-antimicrobial soap and water. When bar soap is used, soap racks that facilitate drainage and small bars of soap should be used.
  - Multiple-use cloth towels of the hanging or roll type are not recommended for use in health care settings.

- Surgical hand antisepsis
  - Remove rings, watches, and bracelets before beginning the surgical hand scrub.
  - Remove debris from underneath fingernails using a nail cleaner under running water.
  - Surgical hand antisepsis using either an antimicrobial soap or an alcohol-based hand rub with persistent activity is recommended before donning sterile gloves when performing surgical procedures.
  - When performing surgical hand antisepsis using an antimicrobial soap, scrub hands and forearms for the length of time recommended by the manufacturer, usually 2 to 6 minutes. Long scrub times (for example, 10 minutes) are not necessary.
  - When using an alcohol-based surgical hand-scrub product with persistent activity, follow the manufacturer's instructions. Before applying the alcohol solution, prewash hands and forearms with a non-antimicrobial soap and dry hands and forearms completely. After application of the alcohol-based product as recommended, allow hands and forearms to dry thoroughly before donning sterile gloves.

(continued on next page)

Figure 2-1: *continued*

- Selection of hand hygiene agents
  - Provide personnel with efficacious hand hygiene products that have low irritancy potential, particularly when these products are used multiple times per shift. This recommendation applies to products used for hand antisepsis before and after patient care in clinical areas and to products used for surgical hand antisepsis by surgical personnel.
  - To maximize acceptance of hand hygiene products by health care workers, solicit input from these employees regarding the feel, fragrance, and skin tolerance of any products under consideration. The cost of hand hygiene products should not be the primary factor influencing product selection.
  - When selecting non-antimicrobial soaps, antimicrobial soaps, or alcohol-based hand rubs, solicit information from manufacturers regarding any known interactions between products used to clean hands, skin care products, and the types of gloves used in the institution.
  - Before making purchasing decisions, evaluate the dispenser systems of various product manufacturers or distributors to ensure that dispensers function adequately and deliver an appropriate volume of product. Do not add soap to a partially empty soap dispenser. This practice of "topping off" dispensers can lead to bacterial contamination of soap.

- Skin care
  - Provide health care workers with hand lotions or creams to minimize the occurrence of irritant contact dermatitis associated with hand antisepsis or hand washing.
  - Solicit information from manufacturers regarding any effects that hand lotions, creams, or alcohol-based hand antiseptics may have on the persistent effects of antimicrobial soaps being used in the institution.

- Other aspects of hand hygiene
  - Do not wear artificial fingernails or extenders when having direct contact with patients at high risk (for example, those in intensive care units or operating rooms).
  - Keep natural nail tips less than 1/4-inch long.
  - Wear gloves when contact with blood or other potentially infectious materials, mucous membranes, and nonintact skin can occur.
  - Remove gloves after caring for a patient. Do not wear the same pair of gloves for the care of more than one patient, and do not wash gloves between uses with different patients.
  - Change gloves during patient care if moving from a contaminated body site to a clean body site.
  - No recommendations can be made regarding wearing rings in health care settings. This is an unresolved issue.

- Healthcare Worker Educational and Motivational Programs recommended by the CDC

  - As part of an overall program to improve hand hygiene practices of health care workers, educate personnel regarding the types of patient care activities that can result in hand contamination and the advantages and disadvantages of various methods used to clean their hands.
  - Monitor health care workers' adherence to recommended hand hygiene practices and provide personnel with information regarding their performance.
  - Encourage patients and their families to remind health care workers to decontaminate their hands.

- Administrative measures recommended by the CDC
  - Make improved hand hygiene adherence an institutional priority and provide appropriate administrative support and financial resources.
  - Implement a multidisciplinary program designed to improve adherence of health personnel to recommended hand hygiene practices.
  - As part of a multidisciplinary program to improve hand hygiene adherence, provide health care workers with a readily accessible alcohol-based hand rub product.
  - To improve hand hygiene adherence among personnel who work in areas in which high work loads and high intensity of patient care are anticipated, make an alcohol-based hand rub available at the entrance to the patient's room or at the bedside, in other convenient locations, and in individual pocket-sized containers to be carried by health care workers.
  - Store supplies of alcohol-based hand rubs in cabinets or areas approved for flammable materials.

- Performance indicators recommended by the CDC for measuring improvements in hand hygiene adherence
  - Periodically monitor and record adherence as the number of hand hygiene episodes performed by personnel per number of hand hygiene opportunities, by ward or by service.
  - Provide feedback to personnel regarding their performance.
  - Monitor the volume of alcohol-based hand rub (or detergent used for hand washing or hand antisepsis) used per 1,000 patient days.
  - Monitor adherence to policies dealing with wearing of artificial nails.
  - When outbreaks of infection occur, assess the adequacy of health care worker hand hygiene.

Source: Centers for Disease Control and Prevention: Guideline for Hand Hygiene in Health-Care Settings: Recommendations of the Healthcare Infection Control Practices Advisory Committee and the HICPAC/SHEA/APIC/IDSA Hand Hygiene Task Force. *MMWR Recomm Rep* 51(RR16), Oct. 25, 2002. http://www.cdc.gov/mmwr/PDF/rr/rr5116.pdf. (accessed Jun. 9, 2009).

solely intellectual nor, given today's generally abundant washing facilities and waterless cleaning agents, practical. It is, to a great extent, behavioral. Many health care professionals have yet to truly internalize the critical nature of the role that physical contact plays in transporting pathogens from person—their person—to person and the persistence of those pathogens in the face of anything less than rigorous personal hygiene practices.

Infection preventionist and EC professionals, accordingly, are working to refine strategies designed to overcome psychological barriers to long-lasting behavioral change, including strategies designed for groups and organizations as a whole, as well as individuals. For example, at the group level, performance feedback on adherence to guidelines, use of work-unit leaders as role models, and efforts to prevent insufficient staffing patterns can all be effective. At the institutional level, targets for improvement include written guidelines, the culture of adherence, administrative leadership, sanction, support, and rewards.

The use of mentoring and role models is especially important, according to Larson. Clinical leaders such as physicians, nurses, or informal leaders set the tone for other caregivers. Seeing these people perform hand washing or hand antisepsis on a regular basis encourages other professionals to follow suit and feel more comfortable speaking up when they notice someone else neglecting such protocols. Because of the complexity of the process of change, single interventions often fail, making multimodal, multidisciplinary strategies more promising, according to experts.

How is your organization doing in terms of compliance with hand hygiene guidelines? Sidebar 2-4 on page 23 presents a hand hygiene checklist that can help in assessing the situation.

EC professionals can be particularly helpful with the technology side of hand hygiene promotion. For example, they can help organizations evaluate, select, and place appropriate hand-washing systems. Current options on the market include features such as the familiar foot pedals to operate faucets and sensor-activated automatic faucets. Systems today make it possible for workers to wash their hands without ever touching a surface. Some systems actually prompt proper hand-washing behavior—for instance, playing a prerecorded voice message over a loudspeaker if someone fails to wash when sensors indicate he or she should based

on computerized data on room exit and entry and toilet use. Other systems use electronic badges to monitor the hand-washing behavior of individuals.

Dispenser Placement

The decision about where to place alcohol-based hand rub dispensers definitely requires EC input. There has been concern regarding hand rubs as a potential fire hazard, but nationwide there have been no reports of fires attributable to or involving dispensers. However, some authorities having jurisdiction might prohibit their placement in egress or exit corridors.

The Joint Commission recommends that alcohol-based hand rub gel dispensers be placed in corridors provided the following conditions are met:

- The corridor width is 6 feet or greater, and dispensers are at least 4 feet apart.
- The dispensers are not installed over or directly adjacent to an ignition source such as an electrical outlet or switch. Adjacent is defined as being at least 6 inches from the center of the dispenser to an ignition source. (Because state or local fire code requirements might differ from the national codes, facilities should first determine requirements for their particular locale).
- In locations with carpeted floor coverings, dispensers installed directly over carpeted surfaces are permitted only in sprinklered smoke compartments.

Several organizations have published interim guidance documents for the placement of dispensers and control of bulk storage of alcohol-based hand cleansers, including the National Association of State Fire Marshals, APIC, and the American Society for Healthcare Engineering. The Joint Commission allowance of alcohol-based hand rub dispensers in corridors reflect the National Fire Protection Association's tentative interim amendment (TIA) presented in Sidebar 2-5 on page 27.

The quantity of replacement alcohol-based hand rub containers stored and used on any floor, including bulk storage in central supply rooms, should not exceed the maximum quantity permitted by the local prevailing building and fire codes. A good example of effective interdisciplinary collaboration in this arena between the infection preventionist and the EC professional is to work together to implement the CDC or WHO guidelines, as follows:

- The infection preventionist works with patient care staff to select the most appealing alcohol-based hand sanitizer and educates staff on its proper use.
- The EC staff help determine the most appropriate fire-safe locations to mount dispensers.
- Environmental services oversees the installation of dispensers, and the IC and EC task force plays a continuing role in assessing usage data to help monitor compliance.

Table 2-1 on page 24 has a comparison chart checklist that organizations can use as a rapid audit of both the WHO and CDC hand hygiene guidelines that are similar to Joint Commission IC requirements.

Sharps Education

The risk of injury from needles and sharps, including disposable needles, over-the-needle catheters, suture needles, lancets, and scalpels, continues to expose health care workers to serious and potentially fatal infections from bloodborne pathogens such as hepatitis B, hepatitis C, or human immunodeficiency virus (HIV). Although precise numbers are not available, the CDC estimates that each year health care workers sustain more than 600,000 injuries involving contaminated needles or sharps, and approximately one-half of these injuries go unreported. Most needlestick injuries involve nursing staff, yet other health care workers also sustain injuries. Fortunately, injuries involving patients are less frequent.

Although needle-less IV delivery systems, needles that retract into a syringe or vacuum tube holder, hinged or sliding shields attached to phlebotomy needles, winged-steel needles, and blood gas needles are among the more recent sharps safety products, the devices are of little value unless health care workers receive training in their proper use and unless they are used consistently across the organization. An organization's safety training should focus on the importance of all employees being alert to the dangers of exposed needles and sharps—not just to themselves, but also to patients. The CDC recommends that health care workers take the following steps to protect themselves and their fellow workers from needlestick injuries[3]:

- Avoid the use of needles where safe and effective alternatives are available.
- Help your employer select and evaluate devices with safety features.

Sidebar 2-3: Hand Washing—Universal Teaching Techniques

- Communicate cross-culturally, using visual more than verbal techniques.
- Consciously model the desired traits and behavior within what are clearly real-life situations.
- Use concrete rather than abstract concepts and examples to illustrate the direct effect on workers, their families, patients, and communities of failure to meet infection prevention and control standards.
- Reinforce personal responsibility.
- Avoid making assumptions about the level of workers' knowledge.
- Use examples of workers solving problems themselves rather than always working under the direction of a supervisor or outside authority.

Source: Adapted from Pyrek K.: Handwashing and cross contamination: Old issue, new approaches. *Infection Control Today,* Mar. 1, 2004. http://www.infectioncontroltoday.com/articles/400/400_431feat2.html (accessed Jan. 9, 2009).

Sidebar 2-4: Hand Hygiene Checklist

- ☐ Are hand hygiene facilities adequate in number and are they used?
- ☐ Does the placement of hand hygiene facilities encourage their use?
- ☐ Are dispensers for alcohol-based hand rubs placed at or near the entrances to appropriate patient and other rooms, as well as in patient rooms?
- ☐ Does the placement of hand rub dispensers conform to applicable local and federal codes?
- ☐ Are hand rub dispensers properly maintained?
- ☐ Do staff know correct hand hygiene techniques?
- ☐ Do staff understand the term standard precautions?
- ☐ Do staff know how to use personal protective equipment, including utility gloves (for environment of care staff)?
- ☐ Does the organization's culture encourage any staff member to remind another to practice hand hygiene if nonadherence is observed?

Table 2-1: Hand Hygiene Checklist for Joint Commission Compliance

World Health Organization (WHO) Hand Hygiene Guideline Recommendations
Comparison with Centers for Disease Control and Prevention (CDC) Guidelines

I. Indications for handwashing and hand antisepsis

Recommendation	CDC Guideline	WHO Guideline	Key Points of WHO Guideline
A. Visible dirt, blood, or body fluids on hands of health care worker (HCW)	A. (IA) Non-antimicrobial or antimicrobial soap and water	A. (IB) Soap and water	Simplifies terminology and does not differentiate between non-antimicrobial and antimicrobial soap, unless specified
B. No visible dirt, blood, or body fluids on hands of HCW in the following clinical situations:	B. (IA) Prefer alcohol hand rub or alternatively, (IB) antimicrobial soap and water	B. (IA) Prefer alcohol hand rub or alternatively, (IB) soap and water	
1. Before direct patient contact	1. (IB) Recommend	1. (IB) Recommend before *and after* contact	Clarifies expanded use of hand hygiene
2. After removing gloves	2. (IB) Recommend	2. (IB) Recommend	
3. Before handling invasive device for insertion	3. (IB) Before donning sterile gloves for central venous catheter insertion; also for insertion of other invasive devices that do not require a surgical procedure using sterile gloves	3. (IB) Before insertion of all invasive devices, regardless of glove use	Clarifies clinical situations and simplify terminology
4. After contact with blood, body fluids, mucous membranes, non-intact skin, and wound dressings	4. (IA) Recommend	4. (IA) Recommend	
5. Moving from contaminated patient body site to clean site during patient care	5. (II) Recommend	5. (IB) Recommend	
6. After contact with inanimate objects or medical equipment close to patient	6. (II) Recommend	6. (IB) Recommend	
C. Potential exposure to spore-forming organisms	C. (II) Non-antimicrobial or antimicrobial soap and water	C. (IB) Soap and water	Alcohol hand rub is ineffective against spore-forming organisms (for example, *Clostridium difficile, Bacillus anthracis*).
D. After using restroom	D. (IB) Non-antimicrobial or antimicrobial soap and water	D. (II) Soap and water	
E. Before handling medication or food	E. (IB) Non-antimicrobial or antimicrobial soap and water (before handling food)	E. (IB) Alcohol rub or soap and water (before handling both medication and food)	Recommends alcohol rub and expands recommendation to include medication
F. Concomitant or sequential use of alcohol rub with soap and water	F. No comment in non-surgical setting. In surgical (operating room) setting, recommend pre-washing hands with soap and water before alcohol rub (*see* **III.G.2**)	F. (II) Not recommended in either non-surgical or surgical setting	Pre-washing hands is not recommended.

II. Hand hygiene technique (non-surgical)

Recommendation	CDC Guideline	WHO Guideline	Key Points of WHO Guideline
A. Alcohol hand hygiene rub	A. (IB) Apply palmful, rub thoroughly until dry. Follow manufacturer's recommendation regarding volume of product to use	A. (IB) Apply palmful, rub thoroughly until dry. See instructional diagram.	Emphasizes hand hygiene technique rather than product volume and refers to diagram
B. Handwashing with soap and water. Wet hands first, wash thoroughly, rinse, dry with disposable towel, and use towel to turn off faucet	B. (IB) Wash for 15 seconds	B. (IB) Wash using vigorous rotational handrubbing technique. No time requirement. See instructional diagram.	Emphasizes hand hygiene technique rather than time requirement and refers to diagram
C. Avoid use of very hot water to decrease risk of dermatitis	C. (IB) Recommend	C. (IB) Recommend	
D. Dry hands thoroughly after hand hygiene	D. Recommend (*see* **II.A** and **II.B**)	D. Recommend; separate emphasis	
E. Avoid using multi-use (cloth) hand towels	E. (II) Recommend	E. (IB) Recommend	Emphasizes CDC recommendation regarding non-reuse of cloth towels by individuals

(continued on next page)

Table 2-1: *continued*

II. Hand hygiene technique (non-surgical) *(continued)*

Recommendation	CDC Guideline	WHO Guideline	Key Points of WHO Guideline
F. Use of antimicrobial-impregnated wipes as hand hygiene alternative	F. (IB) May use as alternative to non-antimicrobial soap and water. Do not use as alternative to antimicrobial soap and water or to alcohol hand rub	F. No comment	
G. Use of bar, liquid, leaf or powder soaps. May use if using non-antimicrobial soap and water. Bar soap should be small size and sit on drainage rack.	G. (II) Recommend	G. (II) Recommend	

III. Surgical hand preparation

Recommendation	CDC Guideline	WHO Guideline	Key Points of WHO Guideline
A. Remove of visible dirt before preparation	A. No comment	A. (II) Wash hands with soap and water	Emphasizes removal of visible dirt prior to surgical preparation
B. Clean fingernails using nail cleaner before preparation	B. (II) Recommend	B. (II) Recommend; clean under running water	
C. Design handwashing sink to minimize splashing	C. No comment	C. (II) Recommend	Recommends evaluating sink design; faulty faucet aerators have been associated with contamination of hand-washing water
D. Remove rings, watches, and bracelets before preparation	D. (II) Recommend	D. (II) Recommend	
E. Artificial nails prohibited	E. Recommend; for high-risk patients (e.g., in intensive-care unit or operating room)	E. (IA) Recommend; for direct contact with all patients	Expands prohibition of artificial nails; associated with changes in normal flora and impede proper hand hygiene
F. Type of surgical hand preparation: either antimicrobial soap and water or sustained activity alcohol rub	F. (IB) Recommend	F. (IB) Recommend; if water quality is not assured, use alcohol rub	Some areas may have water quality problems.
G. Duration and technique of surgical hand preparation			
1. If using antimicrobial soap and water	1. Manufacturer's recommendation; usually 2 to 6 minutes	1. Manufacturer's recommendation; usually 2 to 5 minutes	
2. If using alcohol rub	2. (IB) No time requirement. Pre-wash hands with antimicrobial soap and water.	2. (IB) No time requirement. Apply to dry hands and keep hands and forearms wet during application. Do not pre-wash hands or use alcohol rub and soap and water concomitantly or sequentially.	Pre-washing hands not recommended (*see* I.F)
H. Allow hands to dry thoroughly before gloving.	I. (IB) Recommend	I. (IB) Recommend	

IV. Selection of hand hygiene agents

Recommendation	CDC Guideline	WHO Guideline	Key Points of WHO Guideline
A. Administrative Actions			
1. Provide HCWs with efficacious (effective) product that is less likely to irritate.	1. (IB) Recommend	1. (IB) Recommend	
2. Maximize acceptance and solicit input from HCWs, and include cost as factor in product selection.	2. (IB) Recommend	2. (IB) Recommend	

3. Consult manufacturer's recommendation regarding possible interaction between a) product and gloves, and b) product and creams or lotions.	3. a. (II) Recommend
	   b. (IB) Recommend
		3. a. (II) Recommend
		   b. (IB) Recommend	

B. Dispensers			
1. Access by HCWs: location of dispensers. For alcohol rub: recommend individual pocket-sized containers for HCWs	1. Refers to alcohol rub dispensers only; accessible at entrance to patient's room, at bedside, or other convenient locations.	1. (IB) Refers to both soap and alcohol rub dispensers; accessible at point of care.	Clarifies terminology and encourage flexibility in location
2. Function and deliver specified product volume	2. (II) Recommend	2. (II) Recommend	

(continued on next page)

Table 2-1: *continued*

IV. Selection of hand hygiene agents *(continued)*

Recommendation	CDC Guideline	WHO Guideline	Key Points of WHO Guideline
3. Alcohol rub product dispenser approved for flammable materials	3. (IC) Dispenser not specified but must store dispensers in cabinets approved for flammable materials.	3. (IC) Dispenser must be approved for flammable materials.	Clarifies flammability requirements for individual dispensers
4. Adding soap to partially filled dispensers for refill	4. (IA) Not recommended	4. (IA) Not recommended	Clean soap dispensers thoroughly before refilling to avoid bacterial contamination.
C. Skin Care			
1. Educate HCWs regarding hand hygiene practices that can reduce the risk of contact dermatitis, and provide creams and lotions	1. (IA) Recommend	(IA) Recommend	Provide alternatives for HCWs with allergic or adverse reactions to product

V. Use of gloves

Recommendation	CDC Guideline	WHO Guideline	Key Points of WHO Guideline
A. Gloves are not a substitute for hand hygiene	A. No comment	A. (IB) Recommend	Emphasizes use of hand hygiene after gloves are removed
B. Use gloves before contact with blood and body fluids, mucous membranes and non-intact skin	B. (IC) Recommend	B. (IC) Recommend	
C. Remove gloves after contact with each patient and avoid re-use of gloves	C. (IB) Do not re-use the same gloves (or wash them between uses) with multiple patients.	C. (IB) If re-use is necessary, re-process gloves adequately between patients.	Glove reuse may be necessary in some areas. Recommends implementing a glove reprocessing method to maintain glove integrity while adequately cleaning gloves
D. Change or remove gloves if moving from contaminated to clean patient site or the environment	D. (II) Recommend	D. (II) Recommend	

VI. Other aspects of hand hygiene (non-surgical)

Recommendation	CDC Guideline	WHO Guideline	Key Points of WHO Guideline
A. Use of artificial nails/extenders	A. (IA) Prohibited for high-risk patients, e.g., in intensive care unit or operating room	A. (IA) Prohibited for all direct patient contact in all settings	Prohibition of artificial nails expanded (*see* III.E)
B. Nail length (natural nails); tips must be less than ¼ inch or 0.5 cm in length	B. (II) Recommend	B. (II) Recommend	
C. Wearing of rings in non-surgical health care settings	C. Unresolved issue	C. No comment	

Outcome Measures and Performance Indicators

Recommendation	CDC Guideline	WHO Guideline	Key Points of WHO Guideline
A. Monitoring of hand hygiene compliance			
1. Direct observation with HCW performance feedback; calculate number of hand hygiene episodes performed per number of opportunities.	1. Recommend	1. Recommend	
2. Indirect monitoring			
a. Monitor volume of product used for hand hygiene.	a. Calculate volume used per 1,000 patient-days.	a. Estimate volume used based on nursing activities.	Estimate volume instead of calculating it.
b. Other monitoring	b. No comment	b. Count used paper towels.	Alternative monitoring
c. Electronic monitoring	c. No comment	c. Monitor use of sinks, hand hygiene product or paper towels electronically.	Alternative monitoring
d. Monitor compliance with facility policies regarding jewelry, nail polish, and artificial nails.	d. Recommend non-specific monitoring	d. Monitor compliance by direct and indirect observation, self-assessment and patient assessment	Specific measures to monitor compliance

Source: Joint Commission Resources: CDC/WHO hand hygiene guidelines crosswalk. *Jt Comm Perspect* 5(28):5–8, Feb. 2008.

- Use devices with safety features provided by your employer.
- Avoid recapping needles.
- Plan for safe handling and disposal before beginning any procedure using needles.
- Dispose of used needles promptly in appropriate sharps disposal containers.
- Report all needlestick and other sharps-related injuries promptly to ensure that you receive appropriate follow-up care.
- Tell your employer about hazards from needles that you observe in your work environment.
- Participate in bloodborne pathogen training and follow recommended infection prevention practices, including hepatitis B vaccination.

Beyond safety training, all health care organizations should have a needlestick prevention program in place as part of their compliance with the Occupational Safety and Health Administration (OSHA) existing bloodborne pathogen standard that requires organizations to use safety-engineered sharps and needle-less systems when possible. A successful sharps injury prevention program depends on a combination of safe devices and good work practices. For example, maintenance, IC, and housekeeping personnel should put sharps containers at eye level, near the use area, and replace them regularly.

In its *Preventing Needlestick Injuries in Health Care Settings* publication, the National Institute for Occupational Safety and Health (NIOSH) outlines a number of strategies included in their prevention programs, including the following[3]:

- Eliminate the use of needles when safe and effective alternatives are available.
- Implement the use of devices with safety features and evaluate their use to determine which are most effective and acceptable.
- Analyze needlestick- and sharps-related injuries in your workplace to identify hazards and injury trends.
- Set priorities and strategies for prevention by examining local and national information about risk factors for needlestick injuries and successful intervention efforts.
- Ensure that health care workers are properly trained in the safe use and disposal of needles and sharps.
- Modify work practices that pose a needlestick injury hazard to make them safer.
- Establish procedures for and encourage the reporting and timely follow-up of all needlestick and other sharps-related injuries.
- Evaluate the effectiveness of prevention efforts and provide feedback on performance.

Sidebar 2-5: Guidance on Dispenser Placement

The National Fire Protection Associations (NFPA) tentative interim amendment (TIA) allows the installation of dispensers in the corridors of health care facilities provided the following conditions are met:

- The corridor width is 6 feet or greater, and dispensers are at least 4 feet apart.
- The maximum individual dispenser fluid capacity is 0.32 gallons (1.2 liters) for dispensers in rooms, corridors, and areas open to corridors and 0.53 gallons (2.0 liters) for dispensers in suites of rooms.
- The dispensers are not installed over or directly adjacent to an ignition source (for example, electrical outlets or switches).
- In locations with carpeted floor coverings, dispensers installed directly over carpeted surfaces are permitted only in sprinklered smoke compartments.
- A single smoke compartment may contain no more than an aggregate of 10 gallons (37.8 liters) of alcohol-based hand rub solution in dispensers and a maximum of 5 gallons (18.9 liters) in storage.
- Dispensing units may project no more than 6 inches from the corridor wall, above the handrail height, where minimum corridor width is 6 feet.

The NFPA TIA to NFPA 101® *Life Safety Code®*, 2000 and 2003 editions, is available online at http://www.nfpa.org/PDF/04-4-17FD.pdf?src=nfpa.

- Encourage health care workers to report any hazards from needles they observe in their work environment and to participate in bloodborne pathogen training and follow recommended injury prevention practices, including getting a hepatitis B vaccination.

Even though OSHA's Bloodborne Pathogens Standard requires health care organizations to use—and train workers to use—needle safety devices to fight bloodborne infection, risky practices such as not manually recapping and not properly disposing of needles and sharps are still used regularly, suggesting a need for continual reminders in forms, posters, checklists, staff meetings, in-services, newsletters, table cards, paycheck stuffers, and so on. It should be pointed out that OSHA requires that all sharps injuries be documented in a sharps injury log that contains, at a minimum, the type and brand of device involved and a description of the incident, including the location.

In assessing and enhancing a needlestick prevention program, it's important to look at your organization's needlestick- and sharps-related injury reports to determine the devices most commonly involved, the ways and areas in which injuries occur, and the types of workers most often affected and feature this information in written, oral, video, and computer presentations. As it is estimated that almost half of all needlesticks go unreported, make sure that workers know how and why to report sharps injuries and be sure they feel comfortable doing so—and use those reports to refine your education and training.

Sharps Management

Much emphasis has been placed on the risks of needlesticks and other sharps injuries for clinical staff. However, EC employees, including housekeepers, sanitation workers, and laundry workers, are often the recipients of sharps injuries.

OSHA regulates used sharps as Class II medical devices, and the OSHA Bloodborne Pathogens Standard establishes minimum design performance elements for sharps disposal containers. (Note that unused, discarded sharps are also defined as regulated medical waste.) Such containers should be closable, puncture resistant, leak-proof on the sides and bottom, and labeled or color-coded in accordance with the standard. Of the many available containers, those that an organization selects will depend on its own hazard analysis. That analysis should include the following components:
- Assessment of workplace hazards (biological, physical, chemical, and radiological hazard containment needs)
- Assessment of size and type of sharps to be disposed of
- Assessment of volume of sharps to be disposed of at each point of use
- Assessment of the frequency of sharps disposal container changing and mounting bracket servicing by maintenance staff
- Compliance with federal, state, and local regulations
- Security requirements
- Container transport or mobility needs
- Clinician and procedural variability and movement
- Laboratory equipment variability and movement

- Environmental and disposal constraints
- Economic considerations
- Continued evaluation of medical device technology, including ongoing changes in equipment design and barrier materials

According to NIOSH, it is a good idea to assign responsibility for regular monitoring and maintenance of sharps disposal containers to an individual or group. That person or persons will make sure containers are rendered free of infectious organisms and material each time they are reprocessed and before they are returned to service. In addition, each time a reusable container is returned to service after reprocessing, the facility should confirm that it meets the original performance elements listed in Sidebar 2-6, page 29. For more information on safe disposal of sharps, visit the NIH Web site at http://www.nih.gov.

Staff Training and Education

Those responsible for designing employee orientation and training programs on IC will also want to consult with EC professionals, starting with the organization's safety officer and the plant engineer. Along with IC professionals, the risk manager, and the employee health manager, these professionals can advise on IC-related EC policies and procedures to cover and possibly provide some aspects of training themselves.

Anyone who works in a health care organization might be exposed to infectious pathogens and might, in turn, expose patients and others. This includes biomedical technicians, waste handlers, housekeepers, boiler operators, carpenters, and many other EC workers. Think, for example, of a maintenance person unstopping a drain in a patient room or laboratory. All EC staff should practice some form of standard precautions—including safe work practices, hazard controls, and use of PPE, such as utility gloves, splash shields, and face masks, as appropriate—and all should receive early and ongoing education in the following:
- Disease transmission
- Hand hygiene—why, when, and how
- Standard precautions
- Basic hygiene
- Early recognition of infection problems or symptoms
- Proper use and disposal of sharps
- Proper use of new safety devices
- Handling of regulated medical waste

Joint Orientation and Ongoing Training

The CDC notes that all education in IC should be specifically shaped for individual target audiences and use appropriate examples and language. However, conducting joint orientation to basic IC principles and practices might help to foster the kind of teamwork that maximizes the effect of IC efforts. Most likely, an organization will use some combination of joint and unit- or discipline-specific training.

Most organizations strive to have employees receive orientation before starting work. Make sure all employees receive basic training in IC principles and practices before they have a chance to infect someone or be infected, and provide ongoing training. Here are some strategies hospitals have devised to enhance, monitor, and measure compliance[4]:

- Initial staff education and intervention
- Hand hygiene product measurement and usage reporting
- Patient empowerment
- Behavior modification/change programs
- Visual support materials
- Monitoring and recording adherence to hand hygiene by unit or service (check sheets)
- Providing feedback to workers about performance
- Periodically monitoring volume of alcohol-based hand rub/soap used per unit

Contract Staff Training Requirements

Whether organizations outsource the maintenance of office equipment or the complete job of facilities management, all contracts should spell out IC training requirements. Because orientation and training need to be role-specific, the organization must first identify the services a contract worker or group of workers will provide, where he or she will work, and for how long. The contract worker should then be considered for the same training provided to staff members in a parallel position, particularly if the contract is long term. In fact, contract workers who require the full scope of orientation and training in IC could attend the same program with regular employees.

Sidebar 2-6: NIOSH Performance Criteria for Sharps Disposal Containers

- *Functionality.* Containers should remain functional during their entire usage. They should be disposable, closable, leak resistant on their sides and bottoms, and puncture resistant until final disposal. A sufficient number of sharps disposal containers should be provided. Individual containers should have adequate volume and safe access to the disposal opening. Functional criteria: Consider barrier material performance, closure mechanisms, stability, size and shape, and mounting brackets.

- *Accessibility.* Containers should be accessible to workers who use, maintain, or dispose of sharp devices. Containers should be conveniently placed and (if necessary) portable within the workplace. Accessibility criteria: Consider disposal opening or access mechanism, handles, general location and placement, and installation height.

- *Visibility.* Containers should be plainly visible to the workers who use them. Workers should be able to see the degree to which the container is full, proper warning labels, and color-coding. Visibility criteria: Should carry hazard warning label in accord with Occupational Safety and Health Administration's bloodborne pathogens standard: "These labels shall be fluorescent orange or orange-red or predominantly so, with lettering or symbols in a contrasting

color," and display the biohazard symbol and the word "Biohazard." Red bags or containers may be substituted for labels. Also, consider lighting conditions adequate to display fill status; do not have safety features or security measures distort recognition of container, fill status, warning labels, or opening or access.

- *Accommodation.* Container designs should be accommodating or convenient for the user and the facility and they should be environmentally sound (for example, free of heavy metals and composed of recycled materials). Accommodation also includes ease of storage and assembly and simplicity of operation. Accommodation criteria: Consider worker training requirements, flexibility in design, one-handed disposal, minimal sharp surfaces or cross-infection hazards, simple mounting used only for the specified container. Training could include assembly instructions, safety considerations, maintenance criteria for reusable containers, optimum storage conditions, warranty information, decontamination recommendations, container retirement considerations, bilingual or multilingual material where needed, sharps disposal container disposal considerations, and information for periodic in-service training if required.

A person might need to attend only specified modules of the program. For example, an electrician or plumber working in a defined area for a finite period of time might risk exposure to bloodborne pathogens; if so, he or she should be educated in methods to prevent their transmission in line with Occupational Safety and Health Administration requirements, although this can be done using written materials and training videos along with a posttest instead of a formal class.

In some cases, the organization might choose to make the contractor responsible for providing IC education prior to sending workers out. In that case, the organization might want to provide the contractor with the necessary materials and requirements, or at least review the contractor's materials to ensure that they meet organizational requirements and follow up by observing the workers in action. Some contractors might have extensive experience working with health care settings and might do a fine teaching job on their own, although the organization might still want to provide its own tests to determine that contractors are trained in IC guidelines related to construction projects.

Annual Training

Employees should receive annual training in IC, not only as a means of refreshing knowledge and skills, but also as an opportunity to learn about new developments in the field and in organizational policy. What subjects should an organization's annual IC training program cover? The following list reflects Joint Commission concerns regarding what should be covered in training programs[5]:

- Reporting exposure incidents
- Immunization—guidelines, recommendations, organization policy, and employees' rights
- The importance of personal hygiene
- Policies and procedures for handling regulated medical waste, including who is responsible for various elements of the process
- The role that indoor air quality plays in disease transmission, including the use of special air filters and the difference between positive and negative air flow

Don't forget the "whys," along with the "how"—staff members who understand the reasons for taking precautions and using controls are much more likely to do so. The first IC requirement for employees at Johns Hopkins Hospital is to follow the policies set forth in the policy *Standard Precautions and Infection Control and Prevention Requirements*. This policy covers several of the employment-related issues in the preceding list and is an example of the kind of detail that is appropriate for all employees. It can be downloaded from http://www.hopkinsmedicine.org/heic/policies/pdf/ifc015_Standard.pdf.

Case Study 2-1: Designing for Infection Prevention and Control in the Emergency Department

PeaceHealth's Sacred Heart Medical Center in Riverbend, Oregon was designed with two focuses in mind: To include as much evidence-based design as possible, and to make care processes lean. To the extent that such design contributes to a culture of safety, the long-term process of planning, designing, constructing, and evaluating a new facility has included multiple opportunities for infection prevention and control (IC) improvement. Studies show that hospital–acquired infections (HAIs) can be mitigated by evidenced-based design.[1] To improve the human/system interface by designing better systems and processes, standardization of patient rooms, equipment, and care processes can help reduce staff reliance on memory and includes built-in reminders for performing hand hygiene and/or using personal protective equipment, when necessary.

PeaceHealth began its long-term planning for Sacred Heart Medical Center with making observations and processes leaner fifteen years ago. Functional and space planning began in 2001, construction began in 2005, and staff and patients moved into the new facility in 2008. As staff discovered, the process of examining and designing for increased efficiency and effectiveness of care in any department is long, requiring an interdisciplinary multi-phase process of gathering information and feedback, consulting the best available evidence-based research, and continually looking forward for improvement opportunities.

Observational Stage

Not every facility can afford to redesign or rebuild, but any construction or renovation project requires thorough investigation of current practices before improvements can be made. Therefore, enhancing IC can begin immediately with observations of current facility and design. For example, initial observations with design improvements in mind included the simple act of watching staff perform their daily tasks. During this stage, a repeated observation consisted of nurses interrupting the patient care process to find a thermometer. To pursue the observation to another level, a staff member was assigned to make observations with a timer. Throughout the day, the number of minutes spent looking for a thermometer was added up and quantified in terms of time and dollars lost per day and annually. Every time a caregiver leaves the room for a thermometer or any other medical supply, he or she runs the risk of spreading infection. Particularly, the caregiver will need to perform hand hygiene again, and after having lost time looking for a thermometer, the perceived lack of time may be added disincentive to do so. In this case, human factors—the unavailability of medical equipment needed in the patient room—were negatively affecting IC.

Organization Facts

Sacred Heart Medical Center is one of Oregon's busiest hospitals. Located 110 miles south of Portland, this 432-bed facility is the largest hospital between Portland and San Francisco. Sacred Heart offers a comprehensive range of medical and surgical services, serving as a regional referral center with emphasis in cardiology and cardiovascular surgery, oncology, orthopedics, neonatal intensive care, neurosurgery, spinal cord rehabilitation, and comprehensive psychiatric services.

Project Description

To improve patient care through improved design and the use of human factors engineering in the emergency department.

Outcomes

Emergency department rooms helped improve workflow and used human factors to support healing, add privacy, and reduce the risk of infections.

Case Study 2-1: *continued*

Looking for Solutions

Some identified infection risks—such as the lack of a thermometer in each room and the subsequent chance for failure to comply with hand hygiene—can easily be addressed before moving into a new facility. Other human factors or design issues may take interdisciplinary brainstorming and experimentation. For example, before moving into the new facility staff designed a mock-up room. When the privacy curtain was drawn, it obscured the sink from vision. Unless the caregiver, patient, or patient family member knew the sink was there, it would seem there wasn't a sink in the room. A design that makes performing hand hygiene difficult or seemingly impossible is certainly at odds with IC. Staff wanted to keep the sink where it was, immediately inside the door, but couldn't figure out a way to keep the privacy curtain from obscuring it. Interestingly, it was a patient's family member—and not a staff member—who finally suggested making the curtain straight. Involving a multidisciplinary team—including patients and their families—in identifying human factor problems and solutions was an essential component of the design process. In order to design a physical environment that improved workflow and used human factors to support IC, it was also important to include patients and their families to provide "new eyes" and remind staff of the importance of a patient-centered culture.

IC and Human Factors in Emergency Department Rooms

Although staff was familiar with research indicating that private rooms could promote healing by adding privacy, reducing infection, and reducing transfers, it was decided to also plan for private rooms throughout the emergency department (ED). The decision was made in part because patients indicated they might not share pertinent medical information if they are not in a private room, and because of its potential for decreasing the risk and spread of infection between patients in a shared room, and therefore, organizationwide.

Additional design changes were implemented to improve IC. Each room has two large locked safety glass cabinets containing all "need immediately" linen and supplies. Availability of point of care supplies not only minimizes the number of times a caregiver leaves the room (requiring the need to perform hand hygiene again), it can decrease the number of people entering the room to deliver supplies, and the process of filling the cabinet can be included as part of the facility's process for ensuring medical equipment is sterilized and properly stored. Glove dispensers were included in each patient room, and although the interdisciplinary team initially planned the design with hand sanitizing dispensers broadly distributed, the team eventually decided to limit the dispenser to just inside and outside of each room due to fire rules and to emphasize the importance of hand washing with soap and water rather than relying on hand gels.

Sacred Heart Medical Center incorporated additional human factors designs that don't directly address IC but contribute to an overall culture of safety, minimizing reliance on short-term memory and increasing efficiency—both essential for effective IC. For example, the new ED design includes decentralized work stations between every two rooms, designed at what evidence-based research determined was a comfortable height (39 feet) for standing or sitting at a stool. Electrical outlets are placed higher up on the wall in each room to avoid the need for staff to bend. Ceiling lifts were included in rooms to protect staff from injuries due to patient handling. PeaceHealth staff considered that worker fatigue can increase infection risk, and that taking care of its employees is one way of telling staff that their health and safety is an important part of the care process. Healthy, happy employees are more likely to provide safe care.

Challenges of IC in the Emergency Department

Unlike departments where an acuity-adaptable model of care can allow patients to stay in one bed during their entire stay, there is constant turnover and movement in an ED. Therefore, it can be difficult to track infection transmission in the ED despite the IC improvements that have been made. Currently, Sacred Heart Medical Center does not track infection transmission beyond items like central line insertion in the ED. Although there is an increasing amount of evidence that the environment of care, building, and room design can improve quality and safety, there remains the question of what additional research may be needed to explore the relationship between hospital design and patient outcomes.[1] Particular, IC in the ED after human factors improvements have been made remains a difficult area to track change. One possibility staff have considered is tracking employee exposures to infection in the ED.

Case Study 2-1: *continued*

Designing and Planning for the Future

An efficient and effective IC plan includes anticipating an influx of infectious patients should an outbreak occur and assessing the needs of the community served. Designing an emergency room for flexibility is one way to ensure that the design is minimizing the transmission of infectious diseases (*see* Sidebar 1, below, for examples of flexible designs). To this end, Sacred Heart Medical Center located an imaging/observation area of 12 private rooms designed like the ED rooms and adjacent to the ED. All 48 ED rooms and the 12 observation rooms are essentially the same so that they can be used for any kind of care.

In addition to physical future design, PeaceHealth has joined the Pebble Project—a research program that includes examples of health care organizations with facility designs that are improving the quality of care (http://www. healthdesign.org/research/pebble/). Collaborating with other health care organizations in this way has been part of PeaceHealth's efforts to include rapid-cycle improvement into its future design processes and plans. Particularly in the area of IC and design, it will be essential to continually assess and contribute to a growing body of evidence-based design.

Reference

1. The Joint Commission: Guiding Principles for the Development of the Hospital of the Future. Joint Commission Resources, Oak Brook Terrace, IL, 2008. http://www.jointcommission.org/ NR/rdonlyres/1C9A7079-7A29-4658-B80D-A7DF8771309B/0/Hosptal_Future.pdf (accessed Jun. 10, 2009).

Sidebar 1. Flexible Design

In order to allocate space and resources for potential infectious outbreaks, as well as for potential growth, surges, and technological advances, organizations designing for improved IC should consider the following[1]:

- Master planning strategies—designs with planned zones for future growth

- Loose-fit design—designs with larger spaces that can be used for more than minimum function originally proposed to allow for future adjustments

- Adaptable flexibility—spaces designed to adapt to multiple use (a patient room that can be adapted for different functions, for example, additional rooms with negative or positive-air pressure capacity in case of outbreaks)

- Convertible flexibility—space can be converted for different uses either in emergency situations or when renovating

References

1. Nationwide launch of hand hygiene compliance program for hospitals. Reuters, Jun. 17, 2008. http://www.reuters.com/article/pressRelease/idUS162501+17-Jun-2008+PRN20080617 (accessed Jun. 4, 2009).

2. Boyce J.M., Pittet D.: Centers for Disease Control and Prevention: Guidelines for Hand Hygiene in Health-Care Settings. Recommendations of the Healthcare Infection Control Practices Advisory Committee and the HICPAC/SHEA/APIC/IDSA Hand Hygiene Task Force. MMWR Recomm Rep 51(RR16):1–44, Oct. 25, 2002.

3. National Institute for Occupational Safety and Health: NIOSH Alert: *Preventing Needlestick Injuries in Health Care Settings.* Nov. 1999. http://www.cdc.gov.niosh/pdfs/2000-108.pdf (accessed Jun. 2, 2009).

4. Jaeger T.W., Leaver C.M., Glenn R.: Alcohol-Based Hand Rub Solution—Fire Modeling Analysis Report. American Society for Healthcare Engineering, Aug. 22, 2003. http://www.ashe.org/ashe/codes/handrub/pdfs/analysis_firemodel_final.pdf (accessed Jan. 9, 2009).

5. Trends in health care: Infection control: Zeroing in on infection prevention and control. Health Facilities Management, Dec. 2008. http://www.hfmmagazine.com/hfmmagazine/images/pdf/2008PDFs/08HFMTrends_IC.pdf (accessed Jan. 10, 2009).

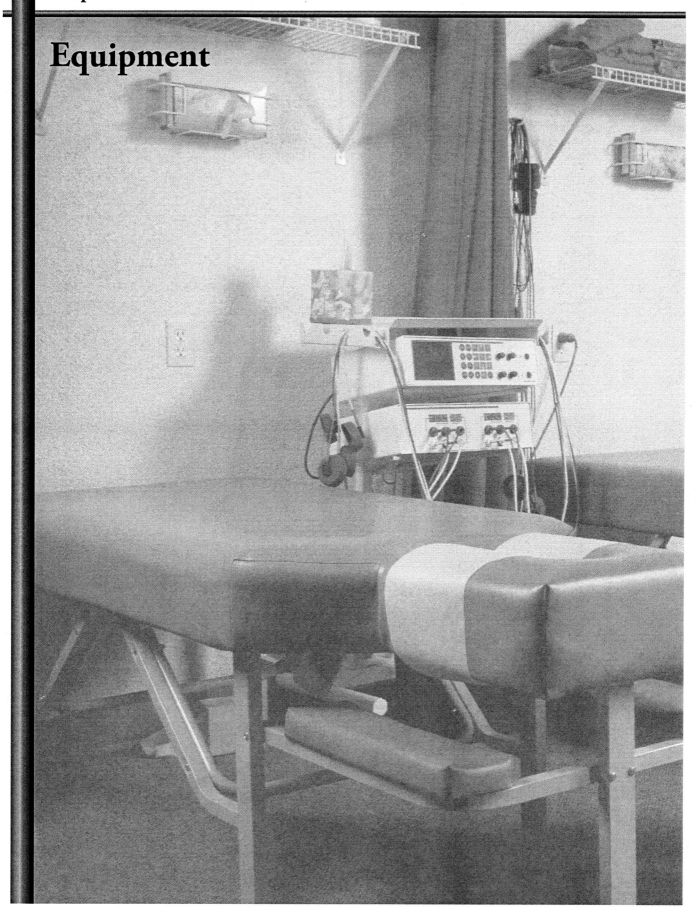

Chapter 3

Equipment

Equipment

Human factors associated with construction and renovation issues that the infection preventionist, environment of care (EC) professionals, and other staff must adhere to were discussed in Chapter 2. This chapter focuses on infection prevention and control (IC) issues related to equipment, including the cleaning of equipment, sterilization, the roles of housekeeping and biomedical engineering departments, and recommendations on reusable equipment, and centralized processing.

Cleaning Methods

Equipment, such as surgical instruments and endoscopes, can transmit infection not only to direct care staff but also to maintenance and repair workers—not to mention care recipients—if not cleaned properly between uses. *Cleaning*, in this context, includes decontaminating and disinfecting equipment. Health care organizations must have policies and procedures in place to address preventive interventions, specifically the following:

- What equipment and supplies can be reprocessed, and which are disposable?
- When should equipment and supplies be cleaned, and how often?
- How should each item be cleaned, including agent and method?

It is up to each organization to answer these questions using a multidisciplinary approach that involves a variety of disciplines including nursing, infection preventionist(s), housekeeping, food service, sterile processing, central supply, environmental services, and biomedical staff. Sidebar 3-1, page 38, lists organizations offering professional guidance in developing an equipment-reprocessing policy.

The Hierarchy of Decontamination

What is sometimes called the hierarchy of decontamination consists of four types of cleaning[1]:

1. *Cleaning*—removes soil and other organic material conducive to growth of microorganisms, usually with water, detergent, and mechanical action
2. *Decontamination*—removes disease-producing organisms

3. *Disinfection*—destroys most disease-producing organisms but not all forms of microbes. There are three levels of disinfection (outlined further in Table 3-1 on page 39):
   - *High level*—germicide; kills all organisms except high levels of bacterial spores
   - *Intermediate level*—chemical germicide registered as a tuberculocide by the Environmental Protection Agency (EPA); kills mycobacteria, most viruses, and bacteria but does not kill bacterial spores
   - *Low level*—chemical germicide registered as a hospital disinfectant by the EPA; kills some viruses and bacteria but cannot be relied on to kill resistant microorganisms (mycobacteria or bacterial spores)
4. *Sterilization*—destroys all forms of microbial life

Which items need which kind of cleaning? Many organizations rely on the Spaulding classification system (or a variation of it) to determine the appropriate cleaning strategy for different categories of equipment.[2] According to the Centers for Disease Control and Prevention (CDC), the following points apply[3]:

- *Critical items require sterilization.* These include items used to enter or contact sterile tissues, such as instruments entering a surgical incision, implants, and needles placed into the vascular system.
- *Semicritical items require high-level disinfection.* These include items that come into contact with nonintact skin or mucous membranes, such as respiratory therapy equipment, anesthesia equipment, and flexible endoscopes.
- *Noncritical items require basic cleaning and low-level decontamination.* These include items that touch only intact skin, such as crutches and blood pressure cuffs.

Table 3-2 and Table 3-3, pages 40-41, present this classification scheme in more detail.

To prevent nosocomial pneumonia, the CDC recommends that organizations use sterile water to rinse nebulization devices and other semicritical respiratory care equipment after they are cleaned and disinfected. An alternative method if sterile water is not available is to rinse with filtered or tap water and then rinse with isopropyl alcohol and dry the item with forced air or in a drying cabinet. Note that only sterile water should be used to fill reservoirs of devices used for nebulization.[4]

Whatever processes, agents, and equipment are to be used, the organization must provide comprehensive and intensive training for all staff members assigned to reprocess equipment and supplies. Questions about high-level disinfectants or how to clean, disinfect, or sterilize a particular medical device should be referred to the organization's infection preventionist, who might need to consult with the manufacturer.

Sterilization and Sterility Assurance

Sterilization is the use of a physical or chemical procedure to destroy all microbial life, including highly resistant bacterial endospores. Typically, hospitals use moist heat by steam autoclave or ethylene oxide gas, or dry heat. However, a variety of chemical germicides are now available that appear to be effective when used according to manufacturers' instructions to reprocess costly reusable medical devices that are heat-sensitive, such as endoscopes.

Sidebar 3-1: Where to Look for Help

Numerous professional organizations provide guidance for health care organizations developing infection prevention and control strategies regarding equipment. This includes specialty groups with their own standards for equipment that their members typically oversee. The list that follows is only a sampling:

- American Gastroenterological Association: http://www.gastro.org

- Infusion Nurses Society: http://www.ins1.org/

- Association of periOperative Registered Nurses: http://www.aorn.org

- Association for Practitioners of Infection Control and Epidemiology: http://www.apic.org

- Federal Drug Administration (FDA), Center for Devices and Radiological Health: http://www.fda.gov/cdrh/

- Association for the Advancement of Medical Instrumentation: http://www.aami.org

- The Society of Gastroenterology Nurses and Associates: http://www.sgna.org

- Society for Healthcare Epidemiology of America: http://www.shea-online.org

---

There are advantages and disadvantages to the different sterilization methods. For example, liquid sterilizers require devices to be immersible. Oxidative formulations, including peracetic acid and hydrogen peroxide, are effective microbicides but can harm rubber and plastics and can corrode copper, brass, bronze, and zinc; instruments made with these materials might suffer cosmetic and structural damage after repeated reprocessing. Sterilization with gas is effective with wrapped instruments (terminal sterilization), whereas chemical methods require unwrapping, so that items need to be used immediately (nonterminal sterilization).[5] Table 3-4, page 42, lists some of the pros and cons to each method of sterilization.

Heat-based methods of sterilization should always be used for heat-stable devices that enter the bloodstream or normally sterile tissues, including accessories to the endoscopic set, such as trocars and operative instruments.

Medical devices that require sterilization or disinfection must be thoroughly cleaned first to reduce any organic material that might interfere with the action of the sterilizing agent. Organizations should carefully follow instructions provided by the manufacturers of both the device and the germicide and should adhere to such cleaning guidelines as the Association of periOperative Registered Nurses' (AORN's) Recommended Practices for Cleaning and Caring for Surgical Instruments and Powered Equipment.[6]

Organizations should also consult the guidelines of the Association for the Advancement of Medical Instrumentation (AAMI), which develops consensus documents regarding the cleaning, disinfection, and sterilization procedures of surgical instruments employed in health care facilities.

Having identified and described the sterilization procedures it will use on the various pieces of equipment in its inventory, an organization must routinely test the effectiveness of those procedures. Biological indicators (BI), available commercially in a variety of formats suitable for the different sterilization processes, provide the highest level of sterility assurance because they test the sterilizer's ability to kill specific strains of highly resistant organisms. AAMI recommends placing a BI inside a test pack to properly challenge the sterilization cycle and testing steam sterilizers daily.[7]

Table 3-1: Spectrum of Activity Achieved by the Main Disinfectants

Level of Disinfection Required	Spectrum of Activity of Disinfectant	Active Ingredients Potentially Capable of Satisfying These Spectra of Activity	Factors Affecting the Efficacy of a Disinfectant
High	Sporicidal Mycobactericidal Virucidal Fungicidal Bactericidal	Peracetic acid Chlorine dioxide Formaldehyde Glutaraldehyde Sodium hypochlorite Stabilized hydrogen peroxide Succinaldehye (succinic aldehyde)	Concentration Contact time Temperature Presence of organic matter pH Presence of calcium or magnesium ions (for example, hardness of the water used for dilution) Formulation of the disinfectant used
Intermediate	Tuberculocidal Virucidal Fungicidal Bactericidal	Phenol derivatives Ethyl and isopropyl alcohols	Same as High
Low	Bactericidal	Quarternary ammonium Amphiprotic amino acids	Same as High
New products introduced on the market often use the same active ingredients as older products.			

Source: World Health Organization: Prevention of Hospital-Acquired Infections: A Practical Guide, 2nd edition. 2002. http://www.who.int/csr/resources/publications/whocdscsreph200212.pdf (accessed Feb. 2, 2009). Used with permission.

This kind of performance testing is an integral part of equipment maintenance. Sterilizers should also undergo the following:

- Daily inspection and cleaning
- Periodic calibration by qualified personnel as specified in the manufacturer's instruction manual
- Periodic preventive maintenance in accordance with manufacturer's instructions
- Scheduled maintenance, including lubrication of appropriate parts and replacement of expandable parts such as steam traps

Maintenance records for each sterilizer should include mode and serial number, date and reason for servicing, and what was done and what parts were used.

Biomedical Engineering

When it comes to IC and biomedical engineering, staff must be aware that all equipment should undergo appropriate cleaning, decontamination, or sterilization before being serviced and again before it returns to the direct care environment. For example, biomedical technicians can feel secure and safe working on a piece of equipment if they know that the system for processing it is effective, practiced consistently, and monitored regularly.

Ensuring that equipment is clean when passing from one department to the next requires a multidisciplinary effort involving biomedical staff, IC professionals, nursing, and central processing. The systems they develop should spell out cleaning procedures in detail and describe how they will be monitored; the procedures should be thoroughly reviewed by each department.

The working relationship between IC and biomedical engineering should be cemented in place with education and training. For example, the facility should do the following:

- Describe the interface in detail, including procedures for equipment cleaning or containment before handoff, during both orientation for new hires and annual training for all staff
- Provide clinical staff being retrained on equipment with a checklist of IC procedures
- Train staff to note the cleaning and decontamination status in the logbooks most organizations keep for checking devices in and out

Education and Training

Although staff who perform cleaning in central services, operating rooms, endoscopy labs, and so on need specialized, detailed training in cleaning and disinfection procedures for equipment,

Table 3-2: Spectrum of Activity Achieved by the Main Disinfectants

	Object: Smooth, Hard Surface	Object: Lens Instruments	Object: Rubber and Polyethylene Tubing and Catheters
Critical items (will enter tissue or vascular system or blood will flow through them)	A, B, C, D, F, G, H	A, B, C, D, F, G, H	A, B, C, D, F, G, H
High-level (semicritical items; will come in contact with mucous membrane or nonintact skin)	D, E, F, H, I, J	D, E, F, H. J	D, E, F, G, H, I, J
Low-level (noncritical items; will come in contact with intact skin)	K, L, M, N, O	N/A	N/A

A. Heat sterilization, including steam or hot air (see manufacturer's recommendations; steam sterilization processing time from 3 to 30 minutes)

B. Ethylene oxide gas (see manufacturer's recommendations; generally 1 to 6 hours processing time plus aeration time of 8 to 12 hours at 50°C to 60°C)

C. Hydrogen peroxide gas plasma (see manufacturer's recommendations for internal diameter and length restrictions; processing time between 45 and 72 minutes)

D. Glutaraldehyde-based formulations (> 2% glutaraldehyde, caution should be exercised with all glutaraldehyde formulations when further in-use dilution is anticipated); glutaraldehyde (1.12%) and 1.93% phenol/phenate. One glutaraldehyde-based product has a high-level disinfection claim of 5 minutes at 35°C.

E. Ortho-phthalaldehyde (OPA) 0.55%

F. Hydrogen peroxide 7.5% (will corrode copper, zinc, and brass)

G. Peracetic acid, concentration variable but 0.2% or greater is sporicidal. Peracetic acid immersion system operates at 50°C–56°C.

H. Hydrogen peroxide (7.35%) and 0.23% peracetic acid; hydrogen peroxide 1% and peracetic acid 0.08% (will corrode metal instruments)

I. Wet pasteurization at 70°C for 30 minutes with detergent cleaning

J. Hypochlorite, single use chlorine generated on-site by electrolyzing saline containing > 650 to 675 active free chlorine; (will corrode metal instruments)

K. Ethyl or isopropyl alcohol (70% to 90%)

L. Sodium hypochlorite (5.25% to 6.15% household bleach diluted 1:500 provides > 100 ppm available chlorine)

M. Phenolic germicidal detergent solution (follow product label for use-dilution)

N. Iodophor germicidal detergent solution (follow product label for use-dilution)

O. Quaternary ammonium germicidal detergent solution (follow product label for use-dilution)

N/A: Not applicable.

Source: Centers for Disease Control and Prevention: Guideline for Disinfection and Sterilization in Healthcare Facilities. 2008. http://www.cdc.gov/ncidod/dhqp/pdf/guidelines/Disinfection_Nov_2008.pdf (accessed Feb. 2, 2009).

Table 3-3: Level of Disinfection/Cleaning Required for Patient Care Equipment: World Health Organization

Application	Spaulding-Classification	Level of Risk	Level of Reprocessing Required	Examples	Storage of Reprocessed Instrument
Entry or penetration into sterile tissue, cavity, or bloodstream. For example, into vascular system, into sterile cavity, into sterile tissue.	Critical	High	**Sterile** Sterilization by steam under pressure or an automated low-temp chemical sterilant system, other liquid chemical sterilant, or ethylene oxide sterilization	Surgical procedure, entry into sterile tissue, arthroscopy, biopsies, intravascular cannulation	Sterility must be maintained. • Packaged items must be allowed to dry before removal from the sterilizer. • The integrity of the wrap must be maintained. • Wraps should act as effective bio-barrier during storage. • Store away from potential environmental contaminants. • Unpackaged sterile items must be used immediately.
Contact with intact nonsterile mucosa or nonintact skin	Semicritical	Medium	**Disinfection** Heat-tolerant items • Steam sterilize where possible. • If unable to steam sterilize–use thermal disinfection. Heat-sensitive items • Low temperature automated chemical sterilant systems • Chemical disinfectant	Respiratory therapy, gastroscopy	Store to protect from environmental contaminants.
Intact skin, no contact with the patient	Noncritical	Low	Items must be cleaned. • Clean after each use with detergent and water. • If disinfection is required follow with appropriate disinfectant, for example, 70% alcohol.	Beds, sinks	Store in a clean dry place.

Source: World Health Organization: Practical Guidelines for Infection Control in Health Care Facilities. 2004. http://www.searo.who.int/LinkFiles/Publications_PracticalguidelinSEAROpub-41.pdf (accessed Feb. 2, 2009). Used with permission.

Table 3-4: Advantages and Disadvantages of Various Sterilization Methods

Sterilization Method	Advantages	Disadvantages
Steam	• Nontoxic to patient, staff, environment • Cycle easy to control and monitor • Rapidly microbicidal • Least affected by organic/inorganic soils among sterilization processes listed • Rapid cycle time • Penetrates medical packing, device lumens	• Deleterious for heat-sensitive instruments • Microsurgical instruments damaged by repeated exposure • May leave instruments wet, causing them to rust • Potential for burns
Hydrogen Peroxide Gas Plasma	• Safe for the environment • Leaves no toxic residuals • Cycle time is 28–75 minutes (varies with model type) and no aeration is necessary. • Used for heat- and moisture-sensitive items since process temperature < 50°C • Simple to operate, install (208 V outlet), and monitor • Compatible with most medical devices • Only requires electrical outlet	• Cellulose (paper), linens, and liquids cannot be processed • Sterilization chamber size from 1.8–9.4 ft total volume (varies with model type) • Some endoscopes or medical devices with long or narrow lumens cannot be processed at this time in the United States (see manufacturer's recommendations for internal diameter and length restrictions). • Requires synthetic packaging (polypropylene wraps, polyolefin pouches) and special container tray • Hydrogen peroxide may be toxic at levels greater than 1 ppm TWA
100% Ethylene Oxide (ETO)	• Penetrates packaging materials, device lumens • Single-dose cartridge and negative-pressure chamber minimize the potential for gas leak and ETO exposure • Simple to operate and monitor • Compatible with most medical materials	• Requires aeration time to remove ETO residue • Sterilization chamber size from 4.0–7.9 ft total volume (varies with model type) • ETO is toxic, a carcinogen, and flammable. • ETO emission regulated by states but catalytic cell removes 99.9% of ETO and converts it to CO_2 and H_2O • ETO cartridges should be stored in flammable liquid storage cabinet • Lengthy cycle/aeration time
ETO Mixtures: 8.6% ETO/91.4% HCFC 8.6% ETO/91.4% HCFC 10% ETO/90% HCFC 8.5% ETO/91.5% CO_2	• Penetrates medical packaging and many plastics • Compatible with most medical materials • Cycle easy to control and monitor	• Some states (for example, CA, NY, MI) require ETO emission reduction of 90%–99.9%. • CFC (inert gas that eliminates explosion hazard) banned in 1995. • Potential hazards to staff and patients • Lengthy cycle/aeration time • ETO is toxic, a carcinogen, and flammable.
Peracetic Acid	• Rapid cycle time (30–45 minutes) • Low temperature (50°C–55°C liquid immersion sterilization • Environmentally friendly by-products • Sterilant flows through endoscope, which facilitates salt, protein, and microbe removal	• Point-of-use system, no sterile storage • Biological indicator may not be suitable for routine monitoring • Used for immersible instruments only • Some material incompatibility (for example, aluminum anodized coating becomes dull) • One scope or a small number of instruments processed in a cycle • Potential for serious eye and skin damage (concentrated solution) with contact

* TWA, time weighted average; CO_2, carbon dioxide; °C, celsius; HCFC, hydrochlorofluorocarbon; CFC, chlorofluorocarbon; v, voltage.

Source: Centers for Disease Control and Prevention: Guideline for Disinfection and Sterilization in Healthcare Facilities. 2008. http://www.cdc.gov/ncidod/

biomedical engineers need basic knowledge of cleaning agents and low-level disinfection. This means the following:

- They can recognize signs of contamination on equipment and know what to do when they detect it.
- They are aware of manufacturers' guidelines for cleaning so they can advise users and central supply personnel on how to avoid damaging equipment.
- They are trained in the appropriate use of gloves and other personal protective equipment (PPE) so they can protect themselves prior to having contact with contaminated items or during cleaning and decontamination.

The same cleaning and monitoring procedures must be applied in equal measure to equipment that is not owned by the organization. Such items should always be cleaned before entering and exiting the organization. Even if the ultimate responsibility for cleaning lies with the contracting company or manufacturer, it is up to the health care organization to monitor the supplier's IC performance under the terms of the contract or an equivalent arrangement. Before drawing up any such contracts, a facility that must outsource equipment repair should seek input from IC and central processing professionals either on its own staff or from appropriate professional organizations.

The Association for Professionals in Infection Control and Epidemiology (APIC) recommends the following CDC interventions to reduce the IC risks surrounding biomedical engineering[3]:

- Clean and decontaminate equipment with approved detergent-germicide before and after maintenance and repair.
- Wear appropriate protective gloves when handling equipment that could inflict cuts or punctures or when contamination is suspected.
- Provide and document training in decontamination procedures, PPE, and procedures to minimize patient and employee exposure during maintenance activities.
- Provide and document employee training in recognizing body substances in equipment requiring repair.
- Work with central sterile supply to assure decontamination of equipment before repair or preventive maintenance.
- Instruct employees in cleanup and disinfection methods before repair, during emergencies, or when normal decontamination personnel are not available.

Reusable Equipment: Reprocess or Discard?

Reprocessing includes cleaning, disinfection, sterilization, repair, reconditioning, and refurbishing of medical devices, either in-house or by third-party processors. Equipment that cannot be cleaned and sterilized or disinfected without altering its physical integrity or function should not be reprocessed. But what about single-use devices (SUDs), which manufacturers say should be discarded without being reprocessed or used a second time?

To many people, the issue is clear-cut: Disposable or single-use devices should not be reused. Period. To others, reprocessing SUDs should be an option as long as it is safe and fiscally responsible. According to the U.S. General Accounting Office (GAO), although SUD reprocessing poses theoretical health risks, clinical evidence shows that certain devices can be reprocessed safely.[8] The GAO reports that approximately 20% to 30% of U.S. hospitals reuse at least one type of SUD. A 2002 survey of surgeons, operating room (OR) nurses, and consumers by the Center for Patient Advocacy found that most surgeons and nurses opposed the use of reprocessed SUDs, whereas most consumers were unaware of the practice.[9]

The AORN states that if the integrity and functionality of a reprocessed SUD cannot be demonstrated and documented as safe for patient care and equal to the original device specifications, the device cannot be reprocessed and reused.[10] But how do you demonstrate that something is safe? At this point, identifying, documenting, and tracking adverse patient outcomes associated with SUDs is not a scientifically reliable process.

Because insufficient data exist regarding the safety of reprocessing SUDs, the FDA announced in 2000 that it would regulate hospitals engaged in reprocessing SUDs in the same way that the agency regulates device manufacturers—*Guidance on Enforcement Priorities for Single-Use Devices Reprocessed by Third Parties and Hospitals* is available at http://www.fda.gov/cdrh/comp/guidance/1168.pdf. That is, hospitals and independent reprocessing firms must obtain the FDA's approval before they can reprocess many devices labeled for single use.

Endoscopes

Endoscopes and similar instruments pose special challenges for IC. Gram-negative bacilli, mycobacteria, fungi, parasites, and viruses will all cling to endoscopes given the right conditions—such as poor manual cleaning, insufficient exposure of surfaces to disinfectants, insufficient rinsing or drying, and improper use of automated reprocessors. Endogenous infections such as cholangitis (from manipulation of an obstructed biliary tract), pneumonia (from aspiration of oral secretions), and endocarditis from bacteremia have also been associated with endoscopes.

Endoscopes fall into the semicritical category; however, if they enter sterile body cavities, they become critical equipment. As such, they should be cleaned, tested for leaks before immersion, sterilized or high-level disinfected with an agent approved by the FDA and according to the manufacturer's instructions, rinsed with sterile water, completely dried, and stored properly.

Staff who carry out this reprocessing should be trained in detail for each specific device they will handle and educated regarding associated hazards. They should be familiar with and have easy access to a spill containment plan for the chemicals they use, including how to assess the situation, what PPE to use, what cleanup supplies to use, and how and when to notify emergency responders.

Reusable Endoscopes

Reusable endoscopes that are not or cannot be properly cleaned and sterilized may be a cause of surgical site infections. Long, narrow shafts are the primary issue, but other design factors complicate the cleaning process: narrow lumens, rough or pitted surfaces, sharp angles, and occluded dead-ends. Modular instruments that are delicate and hard to reassemble invite shortcuts. To deal with these problems, experts suggest that organizations take the following measures:

- Inventory your owned instruments and eliminate those that are damaged, bent, or constructed with inaccessible surfaces that come into contact with patient tissue.
- Compare your policies and procedures with the guidelines on reprocessing instruments from key professional organizations and against the processes that are actually occurring; if they are not up to standard, update them.
- Make sure that staff have the proper tools to carry out the policies, including the right cleaning equipment and solutions placed in an easily accessible location.

- Make sure that staff training in the mechanics of cleaning and managing inventory is designed and conducted by individuals who have themselves been adequately trained and who use a scientific-based teaching protocol.
- Make sure that the number of endoscopes available is adequate for the number of procedures performed.
- Try to keep instruments free of gross debris during procedures; remove any debris that does accumulate immediately afterward by wiping down surfaces and flushing lumens with an enzymatic solution.
- Minimize the length of time between instruments leaving the operative field and the beginning of the cleaning process; proteins in blood and other tissue can dry and cake, making cleaning harder if not impossible.
- Maintain appropriate logs for tracking instruments and their use.

Still, in the end, there is no easy way for facilities to know for sure that an endoscopic instrument can be cleaned effectively, other than to rely on the word of the manufacturer. According to the AORN, a device that cannot be cleaned cannot be reprocessed and reused.[10] This is a good reason to deal only with suppliers of known reputation. Even then, facilities should ask to see documentation that an independent laboratory has performed the testing that proves a device can actually be cleaned of bioburden.

Centralized Processing

The advantages of centralized processing are fairly obvious: efficiency, economy, and safety. Doing most reprocessing in one place allows an organization to more easily standardize and coordinate materials and procedures; more effectively supervise cleaning, maintenance, and sterilization; avoid duplication of infrequently used equipment; and ensure validation and reproducibility of processes. The organization can train one group of workers in technical procedures, thus ensuring a high level of proficiency and freeing up other staff for patient care duties.

To let reprocessing take place elsewhere, even for sound reasons, can stymie the system unless it is coordinated and consistent. For example, at St. Charles Hospital in Port Jefferson, New York, a washer-disinfector was made available in the surgical suite so that gross debris could be removed immediately after a surgical procedure, but nursing personnel sometimes skipped this step and put instruments, unrinsed, right into washer–sterilizers located in the operating rooms. By the time those instruments arrived in central supply (CS) for inspection and assembly, some of them had baked-on protein that made it necessary—and much harder—for workers to reclean and then resterilize them.

To turn this situation around, the organization placed a dedicated central supply (CS) staffer in the OR suite from 9:00 A.M. to 7:00 P.M., Monday through Friday, to handle instrument decontamination on the spot; after the surgical procedure, a scrub nurse prepared the instruments by removing gross soil with sterile water, disassembling those with removable parts, placing them in a mesh-bottomed container, and spraying them with an enzyme spray. Documenting this process and sharing it with both OR and CS personnel ensured that a consistent standard of performance would carry through for on-call or late cases performed after 7:00 P.M. during the week and on weekends. The result was a reduction in instruments that needed to be recleaned or repaired and a faster turnaround of instrument sets for reuse by OR personnel.[11]

Four Areas in Central Processing

Experts recommend that the central processing area be divided into four different areas—cleaning and decontamination, packaging, sterilization, and storage of sterile supplies—with the last two separated by physical barriers. The temperature in all areas should be maintained between 18°C and 22°C, the relative humidity between 35% and 70%, and the airflow directed from clean to relatively soiled areas.

The storage area is not just a place to house products; it is also a means of protecting them against dust, moisture, insects, vermin, and extremes of temperature and humidity, as well as crushing, bending, compressing, and puncturing. Loss of sterility is considered event- rather than time-related, that is, caused and determined by conditions in the storage area and the frequency and methods with which products are handled, as opposed to "use-by" dates. It is a good idea to provide sterile products headed for the OR with an additional dust-protection cover that can be removed before they enter the clean zone.

Certain equipment used on patients who have been placed on central nervous system (CNS) precautions requires special handling and reprocessing because of the heightened danger of infection transmission. Sidebar 3-2 on pages 46-47 shows how one medical center handles CNS precautions. For comprehensive information on this subject, access the World Health Organization Control Guidelines for Transmissable Spongiform Encephalopathies, available online at http://www.who.int/csr/resources/publications/bse/WHO_CDS_CSR_APH_2000_3/en.

Sidebar 3-2: Specifications for Central Nervous System Precautions Transmission Route:
Contact with brain, spinal cord, or eye tissue, cerebrospinal fluid, blood, or other potentially infectious materials

- *Hand washing* is indicated before and after patient contact. Hands also should be washed after removing gloves.

- *Gloves* are indicated if soiling of the hands with blood or other potentially infectious materials is likely.

- *Disposable patient care equipment* should not be reused. It should be discarded into a medical pathological waste (MPW) box.

Sharp equipment, such as lumbar puncture needles, should be discarded into a puncture-resistant container labeled with a biohazard symbol designed specifically for this purpose.

- *Contaminated reusable patient care equipment:* Approval from the hospital infections committee (HIC) is required for reuse of nondisposable equipment that will enter normally sterile tissue, the vascular system, or other parts of the body through which blood will flow. Special processing for these items is required before reuse.

Prior to transport, patient care equipment HIC-approved for reuse should be placed in an Occupational Safety and Health Administration (OSHA) transport tray (a puncture-resistant transport container that has a cover lid and is labeled with "special processing requirements" and a biohazard symbol) found in dirty utility rooms located throughout the clinical center in patient care areas. Under no circumstances should equipment be rinsed, wiped down, or scrubbed. Reaching into an OSHA transport tray to manually handle or remove contaminated equipment is not permitted. Contaminated reusable equipment should be physically contained to prevent environmental contamination (for example, on a procedure tray or in an emesis basin) and safely transported to the soiled (dirty) utility room in an appropriate transport container.

HIC-approved reusable equipment must be reprocessed by either steam sterilization for at least 30 minutes at 132°C in a gravity displacement sterilizer or by a prevacuum sterilizer for 18 minutes at 134°C to 138°C. For HIC-approved critical and semicritical reusable equipment that cannot be autoclaved, such as certain electrodes, immersion in undiluted (1 Normal) sodium hydroxide (which is caustic) for one hour at room temperature followed by steam sterilization for 30 minutes at 121°C is an alternative procedure. Sodium hydroxide is highly corrosive; if use is desired, contact the hospital epidemiology service to make arrangements.*

Contaminated large patient care equipment that cannot be contained in an OSHA transport tray (for example, a bedside commode or hypothermia unit) should be cleaned of visible organic material and disinfected as described by the housekeeping and fabric care department before the equipment is returned.

- Contaminated operating room equipment (including EEG needles and neurosurgical and eye surgery instruments) must be reprocessed by either steam sterilization for at least 30 minutes at 132°C in a gravity displacement sterilizer or by a prevacuum sterilizer for 18 minutes at 134°C to 138°C. Alternatively, these items may be discarded into a puncture-resistant disposable container.

Whenever possible, reuse of contaminated operating room equipment is discouraged.

- *Electronic thermometers* with disposable covers are recommended. Refer to "Techniques for Universal Precautions" for more information.

- *Stethoscopes and blood pressure equipment* generally do not require special precautions. Items contaminated with blood or other potentially infectious materials can be either disinfected with undiluted (1 Normal) sodium hydroxide or undiluted sodium hypochlorite (bleach) at room temperature for 15 minutes or less. Sodium hydroxide is highly corrosive; if use is desired, contact the hospital epidemiology service to make arrangements. Refer to "General Methods for Sterilization and Disinfection" and "Techniques for Universal Precautions" for more information.*

- *Portable monitoring instruments*, such as EKG, ECHO, or X-ray equipment may be used in the patient's room. Any equipment surfaces contaminated with blood or other potentially infectious materials should be disinfected with a hospital-approved disinfectant prior to removal from the patient's room. Refer to "General Methods for Sterilization and Disinfection" for more information.

- *Lab specimens* require special labeling. Label all specimens with a "special processing requirements" sticker.

- *Tissue* requires special handling. A formalin-formic acid procedure is required for inactivating virus infectivity in tissue samples. Specimens must be labeled with a "special processing requirements" sticker, segregated from other autopsy and biopsy tissue, and processed by a laboratory experienced in handling this type of material.

(continued on next page)

Sidebar 3-2: *continued*

- *Patient transport* personnel generally do not need to take special precautions. Transport personnel and personnel in the area to which the patient is being transported should be notified prior to the arrival of the patient so that proper isolation precautions can be taken.

- *Nutrition department tray service staff* provide and remove tray service.

- *Visitors* do not need to follow any special precautions.

- *Environmental cleaning* of rooms should be done according to housekeeping and fabric care department policy. Noncritical patient care items and surfaces (for example, autopsy tables, floors) that have not been involved in disease transmission: These surfaces may be disinfected with either undiluted sodium hypochlorite (bleach). Sodium hydroxides are highly corrosive; if use is desired, contact the hospital epidemiology service to make arrangements.*

- *Disposable gowns* usually are not indicated. However, gowns are indicated in situations in which soiling of exposed skin or clothing with blood or other potentially infectious materials is likely.

- *Masks* usually are not indicated. However, masks are indicated in situations in which splashing of blood or other potentially infectious body material onto the face is likely.

- *Protective eyewear* usually is not indicated. However, protective eyewear, such as goggles or glasses with solid side shields or chin-length face shields, is indicated if splashing blood or other potentially infectious materials onto the face is likely.

- *Personal protective barrier equipment removal* should be done in the anteroom of the isolation room. When the isolation room does not have an anteroom, remove all barriers immediately prior to leaving the room following the procedure described in "Techniques for Barrier Usage." Using the sink inside the room nearest the door, wash hands and, if manual manipulation is needed, a paper towel should be used to turn off the faucets.

- *Private room* usually is not indicated. However, a private room is indicated in situations in which the environment is likely to become contaminated with blood or other potentially infectious materials. For example, a private room would be indicated if the patient has poor hygiene, profuse diarrhea, fecal incontinence, or impaired judgment.

- *Disposable waste and disposable patient care equipment* should not be reused and should be discarded inside the room in a patient waste receptacle lined with plastic. In situations in which the amount of disposable waste generated is such that a patient waste receptacle is not an adequate trash receptor, an MPW box may be kept in the room provided that the following apply: Waste placed into the MPW box is not compacted; the MPW box is closed, secured for removal, and removed from the room when no more than three-fourths full; the MPW box in the room during terminal cleaning is closed, secured for removal, and removed from the room.

- *Clothing, books, magazines, and toys* do not require special handling unless soiled with blood or other potentially infectious materials. Soiled personal clothing should be bagged and sent home to be laundered in hot water with detergent (and chlorine bleach, if practical). If personal items are contaminated with blood or other potentially infectious materials, they should be discarded or disinfected. Refer to "General Methods for Sterilization and Disinfection" and "Techniques for Universal Precautions" for more information.

- *Linen* is placed in a yellow laundry bag with a water-soluble plastic liner.

- *Needles and syringes* should be handled with caution by health care workers. Refer to "Techniques for Universal Precautions" for more information.

- *Urine and feces* should be handled with caution by health care workers. Refer to "Techniques for Universal Precautions" for more information.

- *Handling a body postmortem* requires the same precautions as if the patient were alive. Gloves are indicated if contact with blood or other potentially infectious materials is likely. Gowns are indicated if soiling of exposed skin or clothing with blood or other potentially infectious materials is likely. Masks and protective eyewear usually are not indicated but should be worn if aerosol generation or splashing of blood or other potentially infectious materials onto the face is likely. Label toe tag with a "special processing requirements" sticker before transport to the morgue.

* For appropriate use of undiluted (1Normal) sodium hydroxide or undiluted sodium hypochlorite, refer to current Centers for Disease Control and Prevention *Guidelines for Disinfection and Sterilization in Healthcare Facilities*, 2008, available at http://www.cdc.gov/ncidod/dhqp/pdf/guidelines/Disinfection_Nov_2008.pdf.

References

1. Medical equipment and infection control: Process key in handoff between IC and biomedical engineering. *Environment of Care News* 6(10):1–2, 10, Oct. 2003.

2. Grahs P.: Cleaning and disinfecting: Disinfection of bloodborne pathogens. *Infection Control Today*, Jan. 1, 2001. http://www.infectioncontroltoday.com/articles/410/410_111clean.html (accessed Jun. 2, 2009).

3. Centers for Disease Control and Prevention: Guideline for Disinfection and Sterilization in Healthcare Facilities. 2008. http://www.cdc.gov/ncidod/dhqp/pdf/guidelines/Disinfection_Nov_2008.pdf (accessed Jun. 2, 2009).

4. Healthcare Infection Control Practices Advisory: Guidelines for Preventing Health-Care-Associated Pneumonia, 2003. Recommendations of CDC and the Healthcare Infection Control Practices Advisory Committee. *MMWR Recomm Rep* 53(rr02):1–36, Mar. 26, 2004.

5. Rogers J.V., et al.: Decontamination assessment of Bacilus anthracis, Bacillus subtilis, and Geobaciluss stearothermophilus spores on indoor surfaces using a hydrogen perioxide gas generator. http://www.epa.gov/NHSRC/pubs/paperIndoorBacillus111606.pdf (accessed May 27, 2009).

6. Freeman S.S., et al.: An evidence-based process for evaluating infection control policies. *AORN J* 88(3):489–507, Mar. 2009.

7. Spry C.: Understanding current steam sterilization recommendations and guidelines. *AORN J* 88(4):537–550, Oct. 2008.

8. United States General Accounting Office: Report to Congressional Requesters: Single-Use Medical Devices, 2000. http://www.gao.gov/archive/2000/he00123.pdf (accessed Jun. 3, 2009).

9. World Forum for Hospital Sterile Supply: Subject: Central vs. Local Sterile Service Department. http://www.efhss.com/html/faq/faq.php3?thread+271 (accessed Jun. 3, 2009).

10. Association of Perioperative Registered Nurses: AORN guidance statement: Reuse of single-use devices. *AORN J* 84, Nov. 2006. http://findarticles.com/p/articles/mi_m0FSL/is_/ai_n27072282 (accessed Jun. 3, 2009).

11. Bisol S., Bogue R.: Success story: Centralizing instrument decontamination. *Infection Control Today*, May 1, 2002. http://www.infectioncontroltoday.com/articles/412/412_251success.html (accessed Jun. 2, 2009).

Environmental Services

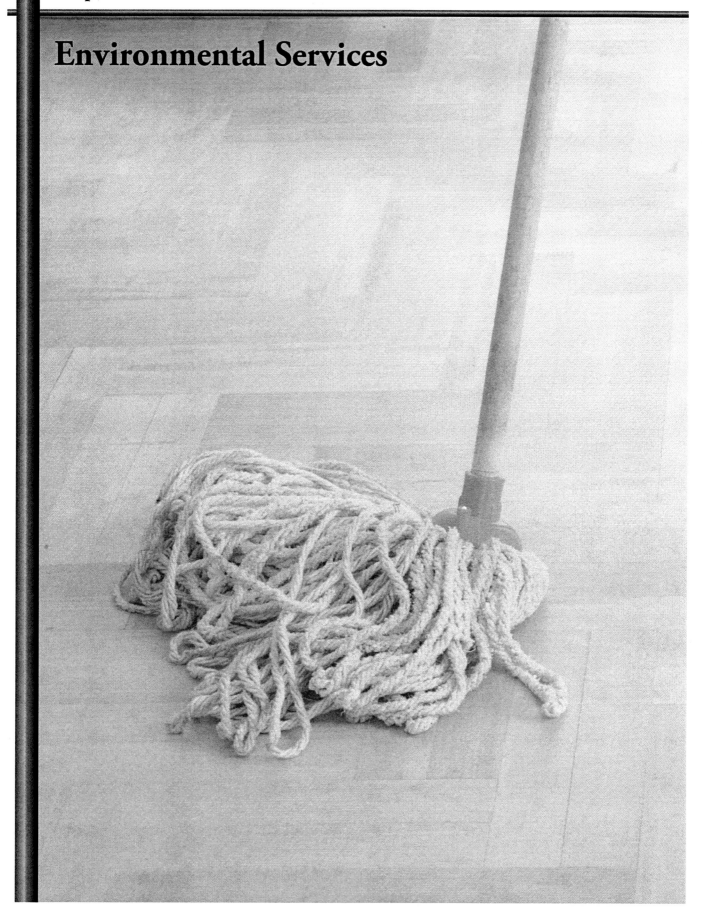

Environmental Services

This chapter takes a look at environmental operations that have an effect on infection prevention and control (IC)—housekeeping and regulated waste disposal. Each function is part of maintaining a safe, infection-free environment, which requires organizations to reduce and control environmental hazards and risks.

Housekeeping

Cleanliness and sterility help control infection in areas that are typically considered part of environmental services (ES), such as housekeeping and laundry. Although The Joint Commission's environment of care (EC) standards do not address these departments specifically, their role in IC is certainly part of maintaining a safe environment. For example, cleaning toys in pediatric units, checking expiration dates of supplies, and reducing the tendency to store things on the floor or under sinks are as much a part of the overall IC program as hand hygiene and sterilizing medical equipment. Indeed, to allow lapses in these processes decreases the effectiveness of the entire program. A checklist for basic IC, presented in Sidebar 4-1 on page 52, suggests the range of commonsense measures that need to complement the clinical aspects of IC.

The experience of health care facilities that have dealt with severe acute respiratory syndrome, which was transmitted despite the use of airborne and contact precautions, suggests that environmental contamination might well play a role in the spread of emerging pathogenss.[1]

Obviously, cleaning patient rooms is particularly important. It might also be the most difficult cleaning job logistically, given the severity of illnesses that inpatients experience; the amount and complexity of medical equipment such as ventilator tubing, electrocardiogram wires, and intravenous (IV) poles that can impede access; privacy issues; the likelihood of recontamination by a health care worker or the patient; and confusion about who is responsible for cleaning what when. Some solutions to these common problems, include the following[2]:

- Use a team approach, getting input from ES, nursing, and IC to define the parameters of the job and determine the best use of personnel.
- Identify which surfaces get contaminated and when this happens most often.
- Determine how often each surface should be cleaned and the methods to be used, including types of disinfectants and cleaning practices.
- Educate workers on the role of the environment in the spread of infection and their role in reducing the risk of this happening, as well as in proper cleaning methods.
- Monitor compliance, including training, appropriate use of the proper type and concentration of disinfectants, and surfaces cleaned.

Fabrics and Inanimate Objects

In addition to patient and treatment rooms, organizations need to have policies and procedures in place to address the cleaning of cooling towers, air ventilation systems, drains, ice machines, carpeting and flooring, elevator shafts, and garbage disposal areas. Some objects and surfaces are more of a risk than others. Gram-negative microorganisms, which can sustain themselves well in very little organic material, are more persistent on horizontal than vertical surfaces and on wet rather than dry surfaces.

Fabric is a special concern. Vancomycin-resistant enterococci (VRE) has been shown to survive for days on upholstered chair cushions in the room of a patient with known VRE, and it was not removed with routine disinfection with quaternary ammonium solution (*see* Sidebar 4-2 on page 53).The problem could be avoided by using a folded sheet or bath blanket on the seat cushion. But a better solution is to use an easily cleanable, nonporous material to cover chairs and sofas in the first place.

All inanimate objects should be cleaned on a regular schedule. This includes the following objects in the following places[3]:
- Waiting rooms (chairs, tables, magazines, and newspapers)

- Restrooms (toilets, sinks—note that too-shallow sinks might harbor bacteria in the drain—faucets, flushing handles, paper towel dispensers, and doors)
- Preoperative and recovery rooms (IV stands, monitoring equipment, beds, and gurneys)
- Nurses stations (computers, keyboards, mouses, monitors, charts, writing instruments, counters, and desk surfaces)

Safety Issues

Thorough cleaning with detergent and water will remove most microorganisms and other contaminants. This cleaning is usually adequate for surfaces and items remote from the patient or in contact with healthy, intact skin. The CDC recommends that organizations not use high-level disinfectants and liquid chemical sterilants on environmental surfaces because these toxic chemicals are not indicated for such use.

All surfaces and equipment that have been in contact with blood or other potentially infectious materials (OPIM) must be decontaminated. However, many grossly contaminated items must be cleaned first with a soap and water solution because the presence of blood interferes with some antimicrobial products.

Sidebar 4-1: Checklist for Basic Infection Prevention and Control for Housekeeping

- ☐ No eating or drinking occurs when care is delivered or where care recipients are seen.
- ☐ Hand-washing areas are equipped with paper towels, trash cans, and appropriate soap.
- ☐ Good housekeeping is performed regularly for dust and odor control.
- ☐ Only approved disinfectants are present on the unit and are used appropriately.
- ☐ Face shields, goggles, and personal protective equipment (PPE) are available and used during procedures and in cleaning.
- ☐ Sharps containers are secured at all times and are changed when three-quarters full.
- ☐ Linen bags are free of holes or tears and are changed when two-thirds full.
- ☐ All items (instruments) transported through the facility are in a closed cart or biohazard bag.
- ☐ All high-level disinfection and sterilization logs are appropriately maintained.

Employee exposure to blood and OPIM is a potential hazard, as defined by the Occupational Safety and Health Administration (OSHA) in its Bloodborne Pathogen Standard (1910.1030), not just in relation to equipment and working surfaces, but also to the following[4]:

- Protective coverings, such as plastic wrap or aluminum foil, should be removed and replaced as soon as possible, when they become overtly contaminated, or at the end of a work shift if they might have been contaminated during the shift.
- Reusable containers, including bins, pails, and cans, should be inspected and decontaminated on a regularly scheduled basis and immediately or as soon as feasible when visibly contaminated.
- Glassware, when broken, should only be picked up with mechanical means, such as a brush and dustpan or tongs, rather than with bare hands.

To prevent contact with blood or OPIM, OSHA requires that organizations develop and implement a written schedule for cleaning and decontamination, based on the following factors[4]:

- Location within the facility
- Type of surfaces to be cleaned
- Type of soil present
- Tasks or procedures to be performed in the area

Cleaning Materials to Use

Cleaning methods used should align with the likelihood of contamination and necessary level of asepsis. Using an ineffective disinfectant, or using an effective disinfectant improperly, can be as harmful as not using a disinfectant at all; all three tactics can lead to patient-to-patient transmission of infection. Different agents will be appropriate in different settings, according to the distribution of clinical isolates with varying susceptibilities to different chemicals. It is up to each organization to specify which disinfectant is to be used in which circumstances from those registered as an antimicrobial product by the U.S. Environmental Protection Agency (EPA) and to follow the EPA-approved label instructions. Sidebar 4-3, page 58, offers more insight on EPA registered disinfectants.

Sidebar 4-2: Limiting the Spread of Infection on Surfaces

Mary G. Lankford, R.N., B.S.N., Northwestern Memorial Hospital, Chicago

Susan Collins, M.T. (A.S.C.P.), Northwestern Memorial Hospital, Chicago

Larry Youngberg, M.T. (A.S.C.P.), Northwestern Memorial Hospital, Chicago

Denise M. Rooney, R.N., B.S.N., Northwestern Memorial Hospital, Chicago

John R. Warren, M.D., Northwestern Memorial Hospital, Chicago, and The Feinberg School of Medicine of Northwestern University, Chicago

Gary A. Noskin, M.D., Northwestern Memorial Hospital, Chicago, and The Feinberg School of Medicine of Northwestern University, Chicago

To investigate the ability of various surfaces to harbor VRE and PSAE, determine recovery of organisms on environmental surfaces after cleaning, and evaluate possible health care provider transmission, 14 environmental surfaces used for upholstery, flooring, and wall coverings were inoculated with VRE and PSAE and assessed for microbial recovery at 24 hours, 72 hours, and 7 days (*see* pages 55–56). Following inoculation, surfaces were cleaned according to manufacturers' recommendations and samples were obtained. To assess surfaces' potential for transmission, healthy human volunteers touched VRE–inoculated surfaces with the palmar (or palm) surfaces of their hands and imprinted their palms onto contact impression plates.

Twenty-four hours following inoculation, all surfaces had recovery of VRE, and 13 (92.9%) of 14 surfaces had persistent growth of PSAE. After cleaning, VRE was recovered from five (35.5%) surfaces and PSAE from four (28.6%) surfaces. Cleaning methods were the least effective in removing bacteria from painted walls, eliminating three $\log_{10}$ of VRE and PSAE. After inoculation followed by palmar contact, VRE was recovered from all 14 surfaces touched.

Many bacteria commonly encountered in hospitals are capable of prolonged survival on environmental surfaces and may promote cross-transmission. Product application and complexity of manufacturers' recommendations for surface disinfection should be considered when selecting materials for health care environments. The recovery of organisms on environmental surfaces, as well as the hands of volunteers, emphasizes the importance of compliance with hand hygiene prior to patient contact.

Acquisition of infections from nosocomial pathogens may cause as many as 90,000 deaths annually.[1] The prolonged survival of organisms, pathogen cross-contamination, and transmission from the hands of health care workers to environmental surfaces and inanimate objects have the

Background

Contaminated environmental surfaces, equipment, and health care workers' hands have been linked to outbreaks of infection due to vancomysin-resistant enterococci (VRE) and Pseudomonas aeruginosa (PSAE). In addition, the structure of certain fibers in textiles and surfaces of building materials such as upholstery, walls, and floors may enhance survival of bacteria, therefore providing infectious reservoirs.

Project Objectives

To investigate the ability of various surfaces to harbor VRE and PSAE, determine recovery of organisms on environmental surfaces after cleaning, and evaluate possible health care provider transmission.

Outcomes

Many bacteria are capable of prolonged survival on surfaces and may promote cross-transmission. Product application and the complexity of manufacturers' recommendations for the surface disinfection should be carefully thought out. The recovery of organisms on environmental surfaces emphasizes the importance of compliance with hand hygiene prior to patient contact.

potential to affect patients, particularly those at high-risk for infections secondary to compromised immune systems. Appropriate disinfection of health care workers' hands, medical equipment, and contaminated health care surfaces continues to be important in prevention of the transmission of microorganisms.[2]

The viability of gram-positive and some gram-negative organisms under various environmental conditions has been

(continued on next page)

Sidebar 4-2: *continued*

previously described.[2,3] Additionally, upholstery materials have been examined for their ability to harbor organisms.[4]

Modes of Transmission

Although it is recognized that the health care environment is abundant with potentially dangerous microorganisms, these microorganisms do not consistently cause health care–associated infections (HAI). Transmission of an illness-producing organism is a complex process. It is dependent on a significant quantity of organism, viability or survival of the offending pathogen, an appropriate method of entry into a patient, and enhanced patient susceptibility.

Health care providers' hands may become transiently colonized with bacteria after patient or equipment contact. Pathogens may then be transmitted from patient to patient through the failure to perform hand hygiene or by inadequate hand-washing technique.[5] Once an organism has reached the patient, it may grow and multiply, causing either active infection or colonization without apparent illness of its host. Patients are a recognized "reservoir" for the transmission of antibiotic-resistant organisms causing infection.

Cleaning Rationale and Disinfectant Agents

Environmental contamination is affected by the amount of activity and individuals in the area, moisture, organic materials that support microorganism growth, and the type of surface. Environmental cleaning necessary for safety requires a thorough evaluation of the extent of contamination, potential infection risk, and the application for surface use. As the health care environment is rapidly recontaminated after cleaning, there is no expectation for the total absence of microorganisms following disinfection in general patient care areas.

Low-level cleaning strategies are recommended for patient care equipment having physical contact with intact skin as well as environmental surfaces not touching patients.[2] Although there is no defined level of disinfection considered optimum for the health care environment, the *Guidelines for Environmental Infection Control in Health-Care Facilities* suggest cleaning of surfaces that is adequate to remove dust and soil to prevent gram-positive cocci, gram-negative-bacilli, and fungus. Decisions regarding the proper selection of cleaning agents such as soap and water, detergents, or disinfectants require information about the surface type and degree of contamination.[1]

Discussion

Our study evaluated various surface materials used in health care environments, as well as the likelihood these surfaces could contaminate the hands of health care workers. We investigated samples' ability to harbor microorganisms and to be adequately disinfected based on manufacturers' recommended cleaning protocols. Results are consistent throughout the three experiments. Additionally, our study suggests there may be a difference in recovery of vancomycin-resistant *Enterococcus faecium* and PSAE over time on these various surfaces. PSAE had significantly less bacterial colony counts at 24 hours, with a reduction relatively consistent over 72 hours. The significance of the difference, however, is unknown. A clinical trial to further evaluate this using human subjects would not be feasible for ethical reasons.

Of note, there were inherent differences between microorganisms used in the experiments. It has been demonstrated that enterococci can thrive in drier environments, whereas PSAE proliferates in moist surroundings and has the ability to develop resistance to disinfectants. These characteristics, as well as obvious designs of the various smooth, porous, or nonporous surfaces, may explain variations among the results obtained. We showed that cleaning could successfully eradicate organisms from many surfaces. Our results, however, suggest that the selection of disinfectants is important for walls and floors. Because repeated contamination of the patient environment occurs, appropriate hand hygiene is important to prevent cross-transmission.

To determine bacterial growth on test surfaces, we reviewed various methods for efficacy, accuracy, and ease of use. These included the swab technique, bioluminescence evaluation, and direct inoculation using an imprint technique methodology. The premoistened swab technique has the ability to directly isolate different microbial populations; however, recovery may not be reproducible or quantitative. The surface rinse approach requires that an entire surface be evaluated. Membrane filtration is also essential to effectively enumerate growth. This methodology was impractical given the size and weight of surfaces tested. The bioluminescence method is not sensitive for low

(continued on next page)

Sidebar 4-2: *continued*

Ability of surfaces to harbor *Pseudomonas aeruginosa* (PSAE) organisms after 24 hours, 72 hours, and 7 days without cleaning, measured by reduction in logs.

Surface	Log_{10} reduction 24 hours	Log_{10} reduction 72 hours	Log_{10} reduction 7 days	Comments
Upholstery				
Woven Crypton®	5	5	5	All upholstery surfaces have reduction in PSAE at 24 hours and continue after 1 week.
Woven solution dyed fabric	4.7	5	5	
Vinyl upholstery	4.4	5	5	
Endurion®	4	4.2	4.7	
Flooring				
Tufted solution dyed carpet with synthetic backing	4.7	4.7	5	All flooring surfaces have reduction in PSAE at 24 hours and continue after 1 week.
Vinyl composition tile	4.7	5	5	
Tufted solution dyed carpet with vinyl backing	4.5	5	5	
Rubber tile flooring with heat welded seams	4.4	5	4.7	
Vinyl sheet goods with heat welded seams	4.2	5	5	
Linoleum with heat welded seams	4	4.4	4.5	
Wall Finish				
Type II microvented/perforated vinyl wallcovering	4.7	5	5	All wall finishes surfaces have reduction in PSAE at 24 hours and continue after 1 week.
Latex paint with eggshell finish	4.3	5	5	
Xorel® wallcovering with paper backing	4.2	4.7	4.7	
Type II vinyl wall covering with nonwoven backing	4.1	5	5	

Common logarithms to base 10 were uses. For example, $10^0 = 1$. $10^1 = 10$. $10^2 = 100$. $10^3 = 1000$. A log reduction of 5 was considered optimal. This was the initial amount of organism that was inoculated onto each of the surfaces.

Source: The Center for Health Design, Concord, CA. Used with permission.

(continued on next page)

Sidebar 4-2: *continued*

Ability of surfaces to harbor vancomycin-resistant enterococci (VRE) organisms after 24 hours, 72 hours, and 7 days without cleaning, measured by log reduction.

Surface	Log_{10} reduction 24 hours	Log_{10} reduction 72 hours	Log_{10} reduction 7 days	Comments
Upholstery				
Vinyl upholstery	3.6	4.0	4.4	Vinyl upholstery is the best performer for reductions of bacterial growth of VRE after 1 week.
Woven Crypton®	2.5	2.9	3.2	
Woven solution dyed fabric	2.5	2.8	3.1	
Endurion®	2.4	NT*	NT*	
Flooring				
Tufted solution dyed carpet with woven synthetic backing	3.2	3.8	3.9	Both carpet surfaces have the best reduction of bacterial growth for VRE after 24 hours. Requires vaildation with another sampling methodology.
Tufted solution dyed carpet with vinyl backing	3.1	3.5	3.7	
Rubber tile flooring with heat welded seams	0	3.1	3.2	Rubber linoleum, and vinyl sheet goods have no reduction in bacterial growth of VRE at 24 hours. Vinyl composition tile continues to have contamincation after 1 week.
Linoleum with heat welded seams	0	2.9	3.0	
Vinyl sheet goods with heat welded seams	0	2.8	2.9	
Vinyl composition tile	0	0	0	
Wall Finish				
Latex paint with eggshell finish	0	0	2.7	None of the wall finishes have reductions in growth after 72 hours.
Type II vinyl wall covering with nonwoven backing	0	0	2.5	
Type II microvented/perforated vinyl wallcovering	0	0	0	Type II microvented/perforated vinyl wall covering and Xorel® wall coverings with paper backing have no reduction in growth of VRE after 1 week.
Xorel® wallcovering with paper backing	0	0	0	

Common logarithms to base 10 were uses. For example, 10^0=1. 10^1=10. 10^2=100. 10^3=1000. A log reduction of 5 was considered optimal. This was the initial amount of organism that was inoculated onto each of the surfaces.

*NT Not tested

For more information on this study and other information provided by The Center for Health Design, visit their Web site at http://www.healthdesign.org.

(continued on next page)

Sidebar 4-2: *continued*

microbial levels and is suitable for microbial counts of 104 to 108. Therefore, direct inoculation by surface-to-agar contact using the imprint technique was chosen for its ease and limited required materials. This involved touching semisolid media plates to test surfaces. Previous studies have shown this methodology to be effective for recovering VRE, *Clostridium difficile*, and methicillin-resistant *Staphylococcus aureus* from the environment.[6]

Although interesting, our results are preliminary, and further investigation is necessary to confirm our findings. Next steps might compare specific hospital protocols to manufacturers' recommendations to evaluate effective disinfection and determine if manufacturers' cleaning protocols require revision. Additional studies simulating multiple episodes of cleaning with these solutions would be useful to measure the ability of various surfaces to withstand disinfection.

In summary, we demonstrated that prolonged bacterial contamination of environmental surfaces encountered in the health care setting is common, especially with environmentally hardy organisms such as VRE. In addition, adherence to the cleaning methodologies described by the manufacturer may not be significantly adequate to completely disinfect surfaces contaminated with bacteria. Finally, once contaminated, environmental surfaces can serve as reservoirs to transmit bacteria to the hands of health care workers. This emphasizes the importance of complying with standard hand hygiene recommendations prior to and following patient contact.

References

1. Burke J.P.: Infection control: A problem for patient safety. *N Engl J Med* 348:651–656, 2003.

2. American Institute of Architects: *Guidelines for Design and Construction of Hospital and Health Care Facilities.* Washington, D.C.: The American Institute of Architects Academy of Architecture for Health Press, 2001, p. 635.

3. Neely A.N., Maley M.P.: Survival of enterococci and staphylococci on hospital fabrics and plastics. *J Clin Microbiol* 38:724–726, 2000.

4. Noskin G.A., et al.: Persistent contamination of fabric-covered furniture by vancomycin-resistant enterococci: Implications for upholstery selection in hospitals. *Am J Infect Control* 28:311–313, 2000.

5. Pittet D.: Compliance with hand disinfection and its impact on hospital-acquired infections. *J Hosp Infect* 48(suppl. A):S40–S46, 2001.

6. Hacek D.M., et al.: Comparison of Rodac imprint method to selective enrichment broth for recovery of vancomycin-resistant enterococci and drug-resistant enterobacteriaceae from environmental services. *J Clin Microbiol* 38:4646–4648, 2000.

Hot Spots

Medical supply carts, janitorial carts, and laundry carts, particularly if they are not cleaned or disinfected between uses, can be of special concern for infection control. Consider a laundry cart that carries dirty linen to the laundry facility and then, without being disinfected, is used to carry clean laundry back to patient care units. Someone touches the cart handles and then touches a patient and, in less than a minute, cross-contamination can occur. In addition, all of the clean linen transported in the contaminated cart is also contaminated.

Carts should be cleaned keeping in mind that many organic soils inactivate sanitizers. It might be necessary to wipe soil off, then apply disinfectant, and then wipe the surfaces down again—taking care not to cross-contaminate the cart by using the first wipe the second time around. This plan takes on particular significance when carts have been near a construction site, where excessive amounts of dust-containing airborne particles might have settled on the surface in a short time.

A problem for many health care organizations is confusion about just who is responsible for cleaning each piece of equipment that goes on each cart. It might be a nurse for certain supply carts, a dietitian for the dietary carts, or a laundry worker for the laundry carts. This is an obvious area for collaboration between EC, IC, and nursing staff.

Another potential trouble spot, ironically, is the hand-washing station. No motivation and technology in the world will keep health care workers from contaminating patients if they themselves become contaminated in the process of washing their hands—by touching a dirty faucet handle with bare hands to turn off the water, for example. Faucets are the greatest problem in this context because gram-negative pathogens cling to wet surfaces with more persistence than to dry ones. Also of concern is the paper towel dispenser because it is the last surface to be touched. This issue makes frequent monitoring of station surfaces a cost-effective strategy.

Finally, think about places where the cleaning supplies are stored. Fungal spores that latch on to cleaning equipment in a poorly maintained janitor's closet can cause that equipment to backfire.

Laundry

Although soiled linen has been identified as a source of large numbers of pathogenic microorganisms, the risk of actual disease transmission appears negligible. Rather than rigid rules and regulation, hygienic and common sense storage and processing of clean and soiled linen are recommended, according to the CDC. Sidebar 4-4 on page 59 provides CDC and National Institute for Occupational Safety and Health (NIOSH) recommendations on this issue.

For example, although commercial laundry facilities often use water temperatures of at least 160°F, the CDC has cited studies showing that lower temperatures can satisfactorily reduce microbial contamination if laundry chemicals suitable for low-temperature washing are used at proper concentrations. Several new detergents are available that have been engineered for this purpose. In fact, new low-temperature, EPA–approved sanitizers now make it possible to sanitize laundry items during the final rinse cycle at just 90°F.

Sidebar 4-3: Information on Environmental Protection Agency Registered Disinfectants

Lists of Environmental Protection agency (EPA)-registered antimicrobial products may be accessed through the EPA at http://www.epa.gov/oppad001/chemregindex.htm. Separate lists itemize products appropriate for use as sterilants, for medical waste treatment, and against the following particular pathogens:

- Mycobacterium species

- HIV-1

- HIV-1 and hepatitis B virus

- Mycobacterium species, HIV-1, and hepatitis B virus

- Hepatitis C virus

Note that products registered as effective against HIV might not be effective against tuberculosis or hepatitis B virus, unless they are so labeled.

The same Web site provides links to quick resources on the definition and regulation of antimicrobial pesticides and on science policy and registration policy documents.

The EPA's antimicrobial hotline is available from 9:00 A.M. to 5:00 P.M. EST, Monday through Friday at the following:

- 703/305-1284

- E-mail: info_anatimicrobial@epa.gov

Similarly, there is no hard and fast rule about when to sort the laundry. Sorting it before washing reduces the potential for recontamination of clean linen that can occur if sorting is done after; it also protects machinery and linen from the effects of objects that might have been left in the linen. On the other hand, sorting after washing minimizes the direct exposure of laundry personnel to infective material in the soiled linen and reduces airborne microbial contamination in the laundry. Again, what's important is that the organization makes a thoughtful decision about this matter and ensures that laundry workers are trained, protected, and held accountable for carrying out the procedure.

In fact, it can be argued that, along with the integrity of the technical procedures used to process soiled linen, the ability and willingness of staff to keep it clean once it leaves the laundry are central to meeting IC objectives.[2] Certainly, safe transport is just as important at the end of the line, when linens have been cleaned, as at the beginning, when it is soiled. This is why some organizations choose to cover laundry carts.

But do the laundry workers responsible for covering those carts and delivering the laundry understand why it is so important? Here is where specialized training comes in to supplement the general IC education that all employees get. One point that sometimes escapes laundry workers and housekeepers is that hand washing is as important for them as for clinical staff, so it is worthwhile to stress the connection and repeat it in newsletters, posters, and department meetings. This plan includes removing soiled gloves and washing hands prior to moving clean linen items from the storage area or cart to the patient room when preparing it for a new occupant.

One IC strategy that some organizations have found helpful is the use of linen packs: an assortment of linen items folded together and shrink-wrapped in the clean processing area to accommodate different tasks that require a consistent set of linens—making an occupied bed, for example, or discharge bed making. Unlike unpackaged items, which must be reprocessed if unused after being stored, wrapped packs can be returned to storage after being wiped off with a disinfectant. On the other hand, assembling the packs can be an expensive proposition, and the wrapping adds to the organization's general waste stream. Linen packs might make most sense where linen storage is far from patient care areas and staff is tempted to hoard items in patient rooms.

Making these kinds of decisions is part of developing an effective IC program for the laundry, which should be a multidisciplinary effort. Organizations may want to pull together IC, nursing, safety, materials management, housekeeping, and other staff along with laundry managers to develop and review appropriate policies and procedures. These might cover the following:

Sidebar 4-4: Centers for Disease Control and Prevention and the National Institute of Occupational Safety and Health Recommendations for Laundry

- Handle soiled linen as little as possible and with minimum agitation to prevent gross microbial contamination of the air and surfaces and of persons handling the linen.

- Bag all soiled linen (if laundry chutes are used) or place it in containers at the location where it was used before transporting; do not sort or rinse it at that location. Covers are not needed on linen hampers for infection control purposes.

- Bag linen that is heavily contaminated with blood or other body fluids and transport in a manner that will prevent leakage.

- Require laundry personnel to wear gloves and other appropriate protective apparel while sorting soiled linen.

To these, the Occupational Safety and Health Administration (OSHA) adds the following advisories, designed to help workers avoid occupational exposure to blood or other potentially infectious materials that might contaminate linens that were improperly labeled or handled:

- Bags and containers used to transport contaminated laundry must be labeled with the biohazard symbol.

- In a facility that uses standard precautions in the handling of all soiled laundry, alternative labeling or color-coding is sufficient if it permits all employees to recognize the containers as requiring compliance with standard precautions.

- Contaminated laundry bags should not be held close to the body or squeezed during transport to avoid punctures from improperly discarded syringes.

- Washing procedures, including chemical formulas, water temperature, wash cycle length, and other technical aspects of the operation
- Employee education and training
- Hand washing—when, where, why, and how
- Sorting
- Transporting soiled and clean linens
- Use of dry cleaning
- Use of gloves and other protective barriers
- Ways of supporting other aspects of the organization's overall IC program

Having input from multiple sources on these issues offers a number of advantages, including the opportunity to collaborate in ways that might otherwise never arise. An example is the development of bed-changing procedures that accommodate the needs of nursing, laundry, and housekeeping staff. An interdisciplinary committee at one health care organization cut patient care costs by documenting for skeptical nurses the successful decontamination of excessively bloody linen—until that time, the hospital had simply discarded such linen. Committees, task forces, or other staff groups charged with developing laundry policies and procedures should consult the CDC Guidelines for Environmental Infection Control in Health-Care Facilities, along with other advisory documents prepared by authorities having jurisdiction (AHJ) and appropriate professional groups.

Regulated Medical Waste Disposal

As part of its responsibility to manage its hazardous materials and waste risks, hospitals are required to establish and implement procedures in response to hazardous material and waste spills or exposures and to minimize risks associated with selecting, handling, storing, transporting, using, and disposing hazardous chemicals. This Joint Commission requirement is in line with the NIOSH Guidelines for Protecting the Safety and Health of Health Care Workers, which call on hospitals to develop a management plan that governs the packaging, storage, treatment, and disposal of regulated medical waste, along with contingency measures for emergency situations and staff training.

Requirements

The first step, according to NIOSH, is to designate the waste that will be managed as regulated medical waste and separate it from the other waste. So what is regulated medical waste? Regulated medical waste can include the following[5]:
- Isolation wastes are generated by patients who are isolated because of certain communicable diseases.

- Cultures and stocks of infectious agents and associated biologicals include specimen cultures from medical and pathological laboratories and cultures and stocks from research and industrial laboratories, as well as discarded live and attenuated vaccines and culture dishes and devices.
- Bulk human blood and blood products
- Pathological wastes are removed from the body during surgery and autopsy.
- Contaminated sharps are hypodermic needles, syringes, Pasteur pipettes, broken glass, and scalpel blades (note that unused, discarded sharps are also defined as regulated medical waste).
- Contaminated carcasses, body parts, and bedding come from animals exposed to pathogens during research, production of biologicals, or in vivo testing of pharmaceuticals.
- Miscellaneous contaminated wastes include soiled dressings, sponges, drapes, drainage sets, and surgical gloves from surgery and autopsies; specimen containers, slides, disposable gloves, and lab coats from laboratories; disposable equipment such as tubing, filters, sheets, towels, gloves, and aprons from dialysis units; and discarded equipment and parts used in patient care, medical and industrial laboratories, research, and the production and testing of pharmaceuticals.

For a full definition of regulated medical waste, see OSHA's bloodborne pathogens standards, 29 CFR.1910.1030. In addition, be sure to consult federal, state, and local regulations to determine if other waste items are considered regulated medical waste.

Disposal Decisions

Treatment and disposal methods include steam sterilization, incineration, thermal inactivation, gas and vapor sterilization, chemical disinfection, and sterilization by irradiation, after which the wastes or their ashes can be discharged into a sanitary sewer system (for liquid or ground-up waste) or buried in sanitary landfills. Organizations should refer to their state or other AHJ for approved treatment methods. Table 4-1, page 61, offers NIOSH's recommended techniques for treatment of infectious wastes.

Certain kinds of medical pathological waste (MPW), such as towels, cultures, and liquid clinical specimens, can be converted to general waste through decontamination or inactivation. The National Institutes of Health (NIH) offers management procedures for safely disposing of such waste at http://orf.od.nih.gov/Environmental+Protection/Waste+Disposal/gen_procedures.htm.

Table 4-1: Recommended Techniques for Treatment of Infectious Wastes*

Type of Infectious Waste	Recommended Treatment Techniques†				
	Steam Sterilization	Incineration	Thermal Inactivation	Chemical Disinfection§	Other
Isolation wastes	X	X			
Cultures and stocks of infectious agents and associated biologicals	X	X	X	X	
Human blood and blood products	X	X		X	X**
Pathological wastes	X††	X			X§§
Contaminated sharps	X	X			
Contaminated animal wastes:					
Carcasses and parts	X††	X			
Bedding		X			

* Taken from U.S. Environment Protection Agency (1986).

† The recommended treatment techniques are those that are most appropriate and are generally in common use; an alternative treatment technique may be used to treat infectious waste if it provides effective treatment.

§ Chemical disinfection is most appropriate for liquids.

** Discharge to the sanitary sewer for treatment in the municipal sewage system (provided that secondary treatment is available).

†† For aesthetic reasons, steam sterilization should be followed by incineration of the treated waste or by grinding with subsequent flushing to the sewer system in accordance with state and local regulations.

§§ Handling by a mortician (burial or cremation).

Source: National Institute for Occupational Safety and Health: Hazardous waste disposal. Chapter 6 in *Guidelines for Protecting the Safety and Health of Health Care Workers.* 1998. http://www.cdc.gov/niosh/hcwold6.html (accessed Feb. 2, 2009).

For the rest of the MPW, however, an organization must make disposal decisions based first on employee safety, but also on the financial and environmental impact on the organization and its community. Do you use a local landfill or must your contaminated waste be hauled out of state? Does your facility provide cold storage for waste before it is removed? What are your state regulations for waste disposal?

Fluid Waste

Fluid waste poses some special challenges. The weight and volume of the suction canister is the most significant item in the contaminated waste stream. Pouring the contents down the drain from suction canisters poses a level of exposure risk that OSHA considers unacceptable. Capping the canisters,

putting them into red bags and having them hauled away by a waste hauler is obviously an expensive proposition, and recent Department of Transportation regulations have added bulk and expense to the packing of infectious fluid waste containers.

In an effort to eliminate the splashing, odors, and aerosolized contents associated with pouring liquid waste into the hopper, facilities have tried many options. One, solidifying the canister contents, poses its own problems: For one thing, infected whole blood that is solidified is not decontaminated, thus sending contaminated waste into landfills. For more information about disposal of infectious fluid wastes, see the NIH Waste Disposal Guide at http://orf.od.nih.gov/Environmental+Protection/Waste+Disposal/.

References

1. Siegel J.D., et al. and the Healthcare Infection Control Practices Advisory Committee: 2007 Guidelines for Isolation Precautions: Preventing Transmission of Infectious Agents in Healthcare Settings, Jun. 2007. http://www.cdc.gov/neidod/dhqp/pdf/isolation2007.pdf (accessed May 28, 2009).

2. McMullen K.M., et al.: Use of hypochlorite solution to decrease rates of Clostridium difficile-associated diarrhea. *Infect Control Hosp Epidemiol* 28:205–207, 2007.

3. Dix K.: Invisible intruders: Inanimate objects' role in nosocomial infection. *Infection Control Today*, Oct. 2003.

4. Occupational Safety and Health Administration: Occupational Safety and Health Standards. http://www.osha.gov/pls/oshaweb/owadisp.show_document?p_table=STANDARDS&p_id=10051#1910.1030(c)(1)(iv)(A) (accessed Jun. 3, 2009).

5. National Institute for Occupational Safety and Health: Hazardious waste disposal. Chapter 6 in Guidelines for Protecting the Safety and Health of Health Care Workers. http://www.cdc.gov/niosh/hcwold6.html (accessed Jun. 2, 2009).

Chapter 5

Utilities

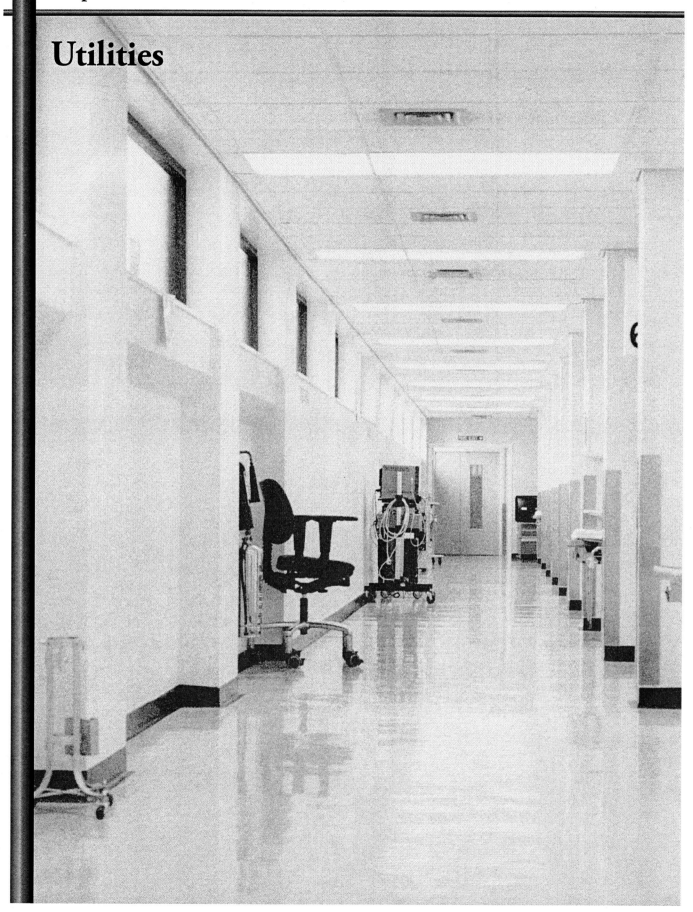

Chapter 5

Utilities

When The Joint Commission emphasizes in the standards that health care organizations should manage risks associated with utility systems, it is referring to at least the following three separate expectations:

1. That the organization ensure the operational reliability of their utility systems

2. That it assesses that reliability and minimizes potential risks of utility system failures

3. That it reduces the potential for health care-acquired illness (HAI) to be transmitted through the utility systems

Specifically, organizations are required to include infection prevention and control (IC) as one of the risk criteria they must address in identifying, evaluating, and creating an inventory of operating components of systems before equipment is used. They must also identify and implement processes to minimize pathogenic biological agents in cooling towers, domestic hot and cold water systems, and other aerosolizing water systems.

The standards also require that organizations document the maintenance of critical components of IC utility systems and equipment for high-risk patients consistent with maintenance strategies identified in the utility management plan and IC principles.

There is no way for health care organizations to successfully accomplish these goals without open communication between the environment of care (EC) and the IC professionals. When working in isolation, neither discipline can be wholly effective in designing, selecting, and maintaining appropriate systems to manage the circulation of air and water so that patients, employees, and visitors are protected from infectious organisms that thrive in these media. This chapter examines the ways in which EC and IC collaborate in maintaining air handling and ventilation systems, air pressure, and water distribution systems that are critical to IC.

Air Handling and Ventilation Systems

In recent years, the simultaneous drop in the number of acute care beds, the reduction in average length of stay, the rise in facilities that provide organ or tissue transplantation, and the increase in immunocompromised patients have put more patients at high risk for often deadly infections. And although the majority of infections are transmitted through personal contact, a significant amount can be either airborne, waterborne, or both. Health care-associated aspergillosis, for example, which is fatal up to 80% of the time in patients with leukemia or HIV, is caused by *Aspergillus* species. "Nosocomial pneumonias caused by waterborne *Pseudomonas aeruginosa* result in approximately 1,400 deaths each year in the United States," reports Matt Freije, a certified water specialist and president of a company that provides consulting and training pertaining to *Legionella* and other waterborne pathogens. "*Legionella bacteria* continue to cause thousands of nosocomial Legionnaires' disease cases each year, not only affecting patients, but resulting in expensive lawsuits, emotional stress, wasted time, and damaging press," states Freije.[1]

Aspergillus grows on cellulose-based materials like gypsum board and ceiling tiles, and its spores easily become airborne once disturbed. Airborne contaminants include other biological agents—bacteria, viruses, and molds—as well as gases, fumes, and dust. The primary means of controlling such contaminants in the health care organization is the design, installation, and maintenance of the heating, ventilation, and air conditioning (HVAC) system.[2]

The Joint Commission recommends that organizations involve design professionals who are appropriately credentialed and who adhere to specifications contained in state and local codes and in guidelines available from the American Society of Heating, Refrigerating and Air-Conditioning Engineers (ASHRAE) and the American Institute of Architects (AIA). These two organizations produce the guidelines that health care organizations historically have consulted in this context, including the AIA's *Guidelines for Design and Construction of Hospital and Health Care Facilities*, 2001 Edition; ASHRAE's *HVAC Design Manual for Hospitals and Clinics*; and the ASHRAE Handbook—*HVAC Applications*. The Handbook's Chapter 7, "Health Care Facilities," has been updated throughout to reflect current guidelines and standards. The Centers for Disease Control and Prevention (CDC) published its *Guidelines for Environmental Infection Control in Health-Care Facilities* in 2003.

HVAC System IC Concerns

From the perspective of these organizations and the Joint Commission, HVAC systems pose the following three areas of IC concern, particularly in areas where immunocompromised individuals are treated or housed:

1. Pressure relationships (whether air flows from corridor to room or vice versa)

2. Air exchange rates (dilution of contaminants)

3. Filtration efficiencies (removal of particulates)

These variables all work together efficiently in an effective environmental IC program. For example, if a patient is suspected of or confirmed as having tuberculosis and is beginning treatment, environmental controls need to provide protection against the spread of infection to others, including staff members and visitors. These environmental controls include local exhaust ventilation, general ventilation, high-efficiency particulate air (HEPA) filtration, and ultraviolet germicidal irradiation (UVGI). The purpose of these controls is to help prevent the spread and reduce the concentration of airborne infectious droplet nuclei. Sidebar 5-1, right, presents a CDC-recommended irradiation approach against tuberculosis.

The particulars of an organization's ventilation policies will depend on what types of procedures it performs, what types of patients/clients/residents it serves, and of course, what kinds of organisms it identifies—different areas might require different levels of temperature, humidity, velocity, and filtration. Air change, filtration, and pressurization parameters for areas requiring special ventilation should be determined through the use of instrumentation. After these settings are appropriately verified, experts recommend that air balancing be done annually to verify engineering controls and before and after the system is modified or breached, as in a renovation.

Sidebar 5-1: Using Ultraviolet Irradiation Against Tuberculosis

Mycobacterium tuberculosis is spread via bacteria-laden droplet nuclei that become airborne when an infected person coughs, sneezes, or even speaks. The Centers for Disease Control and Prevention recommends a combined approach to keep this pathogen from becoming a problem in health care organizations. Many hospitals currently use ultraviolet germicidal irradiation (UVGI) as an auxiliary control measure to ventilation, suspending ultraviolet lamps from the ceiling or in ventilation ducts.

Studies funded by the National Institute for Occupational Safety and Health found that, indeed, ventilation and UVGI worked together to remove or inactivate airborne tuberculosis-like bacteria at a greater rate than either system working alone. The studies also determined that the following measures boost the effectiveness of this technology[3]:

- Increasing the irradiance level of lamps
- Keeping humidity below 75%
- Ensuring that air in the room is mixed

Air Pressure and Infection Prevention and Control

Pressure differential is a measure of air velocity. Pressure control via an offset between supply-air and exhaust-air volumes is essential to keep airborne contaminants from migrating into critical areas. To assure consistent airflow, the offset must be significantly different (with a differential of more than 125 cubic feet per minute for a standard-sized special-ventilation room with less than 0.5 square feet of leakage).[4] Colony-forming units is used to determine the number of viable bacterial cells in a sample per mL. Therefore, it tells the magnitude of infection in humans.

The protective capacity of pressure gradients is more appreciated today, when organizations routinely monitor pressure gradients for system failures or misalignments.

This capacity is particularly significant in special-care units that house or treat individuals highly susceptible to infection due to their immune status or disease processes, such as organ transplant recipients, people undergoing chemotherapy, people with AIDS, and premature infants. These "special ventilation" units, which must be tightly sealed, include the following:

- Operating rooms
- Special procedure rooms
- Delivery rooms
- AII rooms
- Protective environments
- Laboratories
- Sterile supply rooms

EC staff will want to monitor air pressurization in these rooms, which must be well-sealed and supplied with emergency power to ensure continuous operation of ventilation systems, and also to maintain and calibrate sensors and monitoring devices routinely. Table 5-1, below, shows equipment, planning, and evaluation requirements for some of these special ventilation areas.

AIA guidelines permit the use of HEPA filters to clean the air before recirculation as a way to offset the extra energy costs associated with exhausting AII air directly to the outside. The AIA guidelines specify the use of negative air pressure in emergency department (ED) triage and waiting areas and in radiology departments, and positive pressure in outpatient surgery suites when not being used. They also prescribe reversible pressure in isolation rooms and recommend that organizations measure pressure differentials in these rooms, using visual monitoring of airflow into AII rooms and smoke tubes, flutter strips, or other simple devices to measure airflow out of PE rooms.

Recommended Air Exchange Rates

In most locations, health codes allow a reduction in minimum total airflow rates and minimum outdoor airflow rates during unoccupied periods, thus allowing hospitals—which typically occupy only 15% to 20% of their space constantly—to realize

Table 5-1: Areas That Have Special Ventilation Requirements

AT-RISK AREA	EQUIPMENT	PLANNING	ROUTINE EVALUATION
Bone-marrow transplant	Air-handling system: • Filtration • Air exchanges • Positive pressure • Emergency power • Redundant equipment	• Preventive maintenance • Air-quality certification • Emergency planning • Training • Outage notification • Bearings	• Air changes per hr • Pressure differential • Filtration analysis • Vibration check • Fan belts
Operating room	Air-handling system: • Filtration • Air exchanges • Positive pressure • Emergency power	• Preventive maintenance • Air-quality certification • Emergency planning • Training • Outage notification	• Air changes per hr • Pressure differential • Filtration analysis • Vibration check • Fan belts • Bearings
Airborne-infection isolation	Air-handling system: • Negative pressure • Emergency power • Exhaust systems	• Preventive maintenance • Outage notification • Training • Label fan	• Air changes per hr • Pressure differential • Fan belts
Local exhaust areas	Local vacuum system: • Filters • Hose attachments • Air-flow velocity	• Training of operators • Preventive maintenance • Outage notification • Label fan	• Filter changes • Air velocity and/or room-air changes

Source: Streifel A.J.: Health-care IAQ: Guidance for infection control. *HPAC Heating/Piping/Air Conditioning Engineering,* Oct. 2000. http://www.industrialairsolutions.com/contamination-control/hospital-air-purifiers-pdf/HPAC-Indoor-Air-Quality-medical.pdf (accessed Feb. 4, 2009). Used with permission.

significant energy savings by using variable air volume (VAV) tracking systems (*see* Table 5-2, pages 69-70). The AIA and ASHRAE allow ventilation rates to be reduced to 25% of the occupied period rates, as long as continuous directional control and space pressurization is maintained at all times, and the full (occupied) ventilation air change rates can be reestablished at any time.[4]

To determine whether the use of a VAV HVAC system will be effective in your organization, consider the following factors:
- Hours of operation of the spaces being served by the HVAC system
- Magnitude of the difference between the required minimum ventilation air changes per hour (ACH) and the airflow required to meet space-sensible cooling load requirements
- Requirements for continuous directional control: positive, negative, neutral, or no requirement

Spaces often suitable for VAV control include dining areas, outpatient administrative offices, maintenance areas, common areas, and many outpatient therapy areas.

Increased Filtration
Many health care facilities today struggle with staff cutbacks that often affect environmental services. Where this situation exists, it is up to the facility manager and the IC professionals to jointly make the case for spending additional money on HEPA filters or increased air exchanges in areas at the greatest risk and for protection of high-risk patients, as validated by national guidelines and standards.

Filtration is the primary defense against fungi in ventilation systems. HEPA filters might not be necessary; prefilters are effective against most fungi, even when in spore form, provided the filters are tightly installed and well maintained. Keep in mind that fungi can grow in the filters, as well.

Maintenance Needs
Reviewing and approving engineering and maintenance policies and procedures related to inspections and preventive maintenance of utility systems is one of the areas where organizations should get input from both EC and IC professionals.

Fans, coils, belts, and filters all require regular maintenance to function properly. Organizations should establish preventive maintenance, cleaning, and inspection schedules for the HVAC system and should stick to them. It is also important

to keep accurate, up-to-date records of not only routine maintenance but also requested maintenance and quality management activities, including the use of instrumentation to determine appropriate air change, filtration, and pressure parameters for areas requiring special ventilation.

The following are some common maintenance tasks for air distribution systems in health care organizations:
- Change filters when a manometer reading indicates they are full.
- Adjust louvers and dampers for air balance.
- Keep automatic controls in good working order.
- Thoroughly clean ducts if they become contaminated.
- Change pulleys and belts as needed.
- Clean screens and keep them tight.
- Periodically calibrate and test negative pressure alarms.
- Do not allow birds and other creatures to contaminate inlets and other building systems.

Technologies on the Horizon
The most common forms of airborne pathogen control used in health care organizations, but not the only ones, are air filtration, isolation systems, and UVGI. Others include outdoor air purging, electrostatic precipitation, negative air ionization, and vegetation. (Note that the CDC advises using UVGI only in combination with HEPA filters and high rates of purge airflow.) Work on new technologies might provide more effective or economical options in the future. The Graduate School of Architectural Engineering at Pennsylvania State University has identified the following developmental technologies[5]:
- Photocatalytic oxidation
- Air ionization
- Carbon absorption
- Passive solar exposure
- Ultrasonic atomization
- Microwave atomization
- Pulsed light

Sick-Building Syndrome (SBS)
SBS occurs when elements in the indoor air environment affect the health of workers and patients. Proper ventilation and maintenance of a building's HVAC systems are key (*see* Figure 5-1, page 71). John Fishbeck, associate project director in the division of standards and survey methods at the Joint Commission, says, "There are codes that require a certain number of air exchanges per hour in a room, but those codes assume that all conditions are normal. If there is an off-gassing of contaminants from new products during building

Table 5-2: Ventilation Requirements for Areas Affecting Patient Care in Hospital and Outpatient Facilities

Function Space	Pressure Relationship to Adjacent Areas[a]	Minimum Air Changes of Outside Air per Hour[b]	Minimum Total Air Changes per Hour[c]	All Air Exhausted Directly to Outside[m]	Air Recirculated Within Room Units[d]	Relative Humidity,[n] %	Design Temperature,[o] °F
Surgery and Critical Care							
Operating room (recirculating air system)	Positive	5	25	—	No	45 to 55	62 to 80
Operating/surgical cystoscopic rooms[e, p, q]	Positive	5	25	—	No	45 to 55	68 to 73[r]
Delivery room[p]	Positive	5	25	—	No	45 to 55	68 to 73
Recovery room[p]	*	2	6	—	No	45 to 55	75 ± 2
Critical and intensive care	*	2	6	—	No	30 to 60	70 to 75
Newborn intensive care	*	2	6	—	No	30 to 60	72 to 78
Treatment room[s]	*	—	6	—	—	30 to 60	75
Nursery suite	Positive	5	12	—	No	30 to 60	75 to 80
Trauma room[f, s]	Positive	5	12	—	No	45 to 55	62 to 80
Anesthesia gas storage	Negative	—	8	Yes	—	—	—
GI Endoscopy	Negative	2	6	—	No	30 to 60	68 to 73
Bronchoscopy[q]	Negative	2	12	Yes	No	30 to 60	68 to 73
Emergency waiting rooms	Negative	2	12	Yes	—	30 to 60	74 ± 2
Triage	Negative	2	12	Yes	—	—	70 to 75
Radiology waiting rooms	Negative	2	12	Yes[t, u]	—	—	70 to 75
Nursing							
Patient room	*	2	6[v]	—	—	30 (W), 50 (S)	75 ± 2
Toilet room[g]	Negative	Optional	10	Yes	No	—	—
Newborn nursery suite	*	2	6	—	No	30 to 60	72 to 78
Protective environment room[i, q, w]	Positive	2	12	—	No	—	75
Airborne infection isolation room[h, q, x]	Negative	2	12	Yes[u]	No	—	75
Isolation alcove or anteroom[w, x]	Pos./Neg.	2	10	Yes	No	—	—
Labor/delivery/recovery/postpartum (LDRP)	*	2	6[v]	—	—	30 (W), 50 (S)	75 ± 2
Public corridor	Negative	2	2	—	—	—	—
Patient corridor	*	2	4	—	—	—	—
Ancillary							
Radiology[y]							
X-ray (diagnostic and treatment)	*	2	6	—	—	40 (W), 50 (S)	78 to 80
X-ray (surgery/critical care and catheterization)	Positive	3	15	—	No	30 to 60	70 to 75
Darkroom	Negative	2	10	Yes[j]	No	—	—
Laboratory, general[y]	Negative	2	6	Yes	No	30 to 60	74 ± 2
Laboratory, bacteriology	Negative	2	6	Yes	No	30 to 60	74 ± 2
Laboratory, biochemistry[y]	Positive	2	6	—	No	30 to 60	74 ± 2
Laboratory, cytology	Negative	2	6	Yes	No	30 to 60	74 ± 2
Laboratory, glasswashing	Negative	Optional	10	Yes	—	—	—
Laboratory, histology	Negative	2	6	Yes	No	30 to 60	74 ± 2
Microbiology[y]	Negative	—	6	Yes	No	30 to 60	74 ± 2
Laboratory, nuclear medicine	Negative	2	6	Yes	No	30 to 60	74 ± 2
Laboratory, pathology	Negative	2	6	Yes	No	30 to 60	74 ± 2
Laboratory, serology	Positive	2	6	Yes	No	30 to 60	74 ± 2
Laboratory, sterilizing	Negative	Optional	10	Yes	No	30 to 60	74 ± 2
Laboratory, media transfer	Positive	2	4	—	No	30 to 60	74 ± 2
Autopsy room[q]	Negative	2	12	Yes	No	—	—
Nonrefrigerated body-holding room[k]	Negative	Optional	10	Yes	No	—	70
Pharmacy	Positive	2	4	—	—	30 to 60	74 ± 2
Administration							
Admitting and Waiting Rooms	Negative	2	6	Yes	—	30 to 60	74 ± 2
Diagnostic and Treatment							
Bronchoscopy, sputum collection, and pentamidine administration	Negative	2	12	Yes	—	30 to 60	74 ± 2
Examination room	*	2	6	—	—	30 to 60	74 ± 2
Medication room	Positive	2	4	—	—	30 to 60	74 ± 2
Treatment room	*	2	6	—	—	30 (W), 50 (S)	75 ± 2
Physical therapy and hydrotherapy	Negative	2	6	—	—	30 to 60	72 to 78/up to 80
Soiled workroom or soiled holding	Negative	2	10	Yes	No	30 to 60	72 to 78
Clean workroom or clean holding	Positive	2	4	—	—	—	—
Sterilizing and Supply							
ETO-sterilizer room	Negative	—	10	Yes	No	30 to 60	72 to 78
Sterilizer equipment room	Negative	—	10	Yes	No	30 to 60	74 ± 2
Central medical and surgical supply							
Soiled or decontamination room	Negative	2	6	Yes	No	30 to 60	72 to 78
Clean workroom	Positive	2	4	—	No	30 to 60	72 to 78
Sterile storage	Positive	2	4	—	—	Under 50	74 ± 2

(continued on next page)

Table 5-2: *continued*

Function Space	Pressure Relationship to Adjacent Areas[a]	Minimum Air Changes of Outside Air per Hour[b]	Minimum Total Air Changes per Hour[c]	All Air Exhausted Directly to Outside[m]	Air Recirculated Within Room Units[d]	Relative Humidity,[n] %	Design Temperature,[o] °F
Service							
Food preparation center[l]	*	2	10	Yes	No	—	—
Warewashing	Negative	Optional	10	Yes	No	—	—
Dietary day storage	*	Optional	2	—	No	—	—
Laundry, general	Negative	2	10	Yes	No	—	—
Soiled linen sorting and storage	Negative	Optional	10	Yes	No	—	—
Clean linen storage	Positive	2 (Optional)	2	—	—	—	—
Linen and trash chute room	Negative	Optional	10	Yes	No	—	—
Bedpan room	Negative	Optional	10	Yes	No	—	—
Bathroom	Negative	Optional	10	Yes	No	—	72 to 78
Janitor's closet	Negative	Optional	10	Yes	No	—	—

(W) = winter   (S) = summer   * = Continuous directional control not required

[a] Where continuous directional control is not required, variations should be minimized; in no case should a lack of directional control allow spread of infection from one area to another. Boundaries between functional areas (wards or departments) should have directional control. Lewis (1988) describes ways to maintain directional control by applying air-tracking controls. Ventilation system design should provide air movement, generally from clean to less clean areas. If any VAV or load-shedding system is used for energy conservation, it must not compromise pressure-balancing relationships or minimum air changes required by the table. See note z for additional information.

[b] Ventilation rates in this table cover ventilation for comfort, as well as for asepsis and odor control in areas of acute-care hospitals that directly affect patient care. Ventilation rates in accordance with ASHRAE *Standard* 62, Ventilation for Acceptable Indoor Air Quality, should be used for areas for which specific ventilation rates are not given. Where a higher outside air requirement is called for in *Standard* 62 than here, use the higher value.

[c] Total air changes indicated should be either supplied or, where required, exhausted. Number of air changes can be reduced when the room is unoccupied, if the pressure relationship is maintained and the number of air changes indicated is reestablished any time the space is used. Air changes shown are minimum values. Higher values should be used when required to maintain room temperature and humidity conditions based on the cooling load of the space (lights, equipment, people, exterior walls and windows, etc.).

[d] Recirculating HEPA filter units used for infection control (without heating or cooling coils) are acceptable. Gravity-type heating or cooling units such as radiators or convectors should not be used in operating rooms and other special-care areas.

[e] For operating rooms, 100% outside air should be used only when codes require it and only if heat recovery devices are used.

[f] "Trauma room" here is a first-aid room and/or emergency room used for general initial treatment of accident victims. The operating room in the trauma center that is routinely used for emergency surgery should be treated as an operating room.

[g] See section on Patient Rooms for discussion of central toilet exhaust system design.

[h] "Airborne infectious isolation rooms" here are those that might be used for infectious patients in the average community hospital. The rooms are negatively pressurized. Some may have a separate anteroom. See the section on Infectious Isolation Unit for more information.

[i] Protective-environment rooms are those used for immunosuppressed patients, positively pressurized to protect the patient. Anterooms are generally required and should be negatively pressurized with respect to the patient room.

[j] All air need not be exhausted if darkroom equipment has scavenging exhaust duct attached and meets ventilation standards of NIOSH, OSHA, and local employee exposure limits.

[k] A nonrefrigerated body-holding room is only applicable to facilities that do not perform autopsies onsite and use the space for short periods while waiting for the body to be transferred.

[l] Food preparation centers should have an excess of air supply for positive pressurization when hoods are not in operation. The number of air changes may be reduced or varied for odor control when the space is not in use. Minimum total air changes per hour should be that required to provide proper makeup air to kitchen exhaust systems. (See Chapter 31, Kitchen Ventilation.) Also, exfiltration or infiltration to or from exit corridors must not compromise exit corridor restrictions of NFPA *Standard* 90A, pressure requirements of NFPA *Standard* 96, or the maximum defined in the table. The number of air changes may be reduced or varied as required for odor control when the space is not in use. See AIA (2001), Section 7.31.D1.p.

[m] Areas with contamination and/or odor problems should be exhausted to the outside and not recirculated to other areas. Individual circumstances may require special consideration for air exhaust to the outside (e.g., intensive care units where patients with pulmonary infection are treated, rooms for burn patients). To satisfy exhaust needs, replacement air from the outside is necessary. Minimum outside air quantities should remain constant while the system is in operation.

[n] Relative humidity ranges listed are minimum and maximum limits where control is specifically needed. These limits are not intended to be independent of space temperature. For example, relative humidity is expected to be at the higher end of the range when the temperature is also at the higher end, and vice versa.

[o] For indicated temperature ranges, systems should be capable of maintaining the rooms at any point within the range during normal operation. A single figure indicates a heating or cooling capacity to at least meet the indicated temperature. This is usually applicable when patients may be undressed and require a warmer environment. Use of lower temperature is acceptable when patients' comfort and medical conditions require those conditions.

[p] NIOSH *Criteria Documents* 75-137 and 96-107 on waste anesthetic gases and nitrous oxide indicate a need for both local exhaust (scavenging) systems and general ventilation of areas in which these gases are used.

[q] Differential pressure between space and corridors should be a minimum of 0.01 in. of water. If monitoring device alarms are installed, allowances should be made to prevent nuisance alarms.

[r] Because some surgeons or surgical procedures may require room temperatures outside the indicated range, operating room design conditions should be developed in consort with all users, surgeons, anesthesiologists, and nursing staff.

[s] The first-aid and/or emergency room used for initial treatment of accident victims can be ventilated as for the treatment room. Treatment rooms used for cryosurgery with nitrous oxide should have provisions for exhausting waste gases.

[t] In a recirculating ventilation system, HEPA filters can be used instead of exhausting the air to the outside; return air should pass through the HEPA filters before being introduced to any other spaces.

[u] If exhausting air from an airborne-infection isolation room to the outside is not practical, the air may be returned through HEPA filters to the air-handling system exclusively serving the isolation room.

[v] Total air changes per room for patient rooms, and labor/delivery/recovery/postpartum rooms may be reduced to four when using supplemental heating and/or cooling systems (radiant heating and cooling, baseboard heating, etc.).

[w] Protective-environment airflow design specifications protect the patient from common environmental airborne infectious microbes (e.g., *Aspergillus* spores). They should provide directed airflow from the cleanest patient area to less clean areas. HEPA filters at 99.9% efficiency to 0.3 μm should be used in the supply airstream, to protect patient rooms from environmental microbes in ventilation system components. Recirculation HEPA filters can be used to increase equivalent room air exchanges. Constant-volume airflow is required for consistent ventilation. If design criteria indicate that airborne-infection isolation is necessary for protective-environment patients, an anteroom should be provided. Rooms with reversible airflow provisions (to allow switching between protective-environment and airborne-infection isolation) are not acceptable (AIA 2001).

[x] "Infectious disease isolation (AII) room" here is one used to isolate the airborne spread of infectious diseases, such as measles, varicella, or tuberculosis. Design should include provision for normal patient care during periods not requiring isolation. Supplemental recirculating devices may be used in the patient room to increase the equivalent room air exchanges; however, they do not provide outside air requirements. Air may be recirculated within individual isolation rooms if HEPA filters are used. Rooms with reversible airflow provisions (to allow switching between protective-environment and AII) are not acceptable (AIA 2001).

[y] When required, provide appropriate hoods and exhaust devices for noxious gases or vapors (AIA (2001), see Section 7.31.D14 and 7.31.D15, and NFPA *Standard* 99).

[z] Simple visual methods such as smoke trail, ball-in-tube, or flutterstrip can be used to verify airflow direction. These devices require a minimum differential air pressure to indicate airflow direction. Per AIA (2001) guidelines, recirculating devices with HEPA filters may be used in existing facilities as interim, supplemental environmental controls to meet requirements for airborne infectious agents control. Design limitations must be recognized. Either portable or fixed systems should prevent stagnation and short-circuiting of airflow. Supply and exhaust locations should direct clean air to work areas across the infectious source, and then to the exhaust, so that health care workers are not positioned between the infectious source and the exhaust. Systems design should also allow easy access for scheduled preventative maintenance and cleaning.

Source: American Society of Heating, Refrigerating and Air-Conditioning Engineers: *2003 ASHRAE Applications Handbook.* 2003. http://www.ashrae.org. Used with permission.

Figure 5-1: Sample Indoor Air Quality Maintenance Checklist

Building:_____ A/C System: _____ Date: _____

Technician:_____ Signature: _____

Component or Element	Action or Comment
Unit Casing: All sections are airtight and clean inside; all access panels are secured	
Outside Air Section: Check for any obstructions at louver and proper damper operation.	
Mixing Plenum: Proper damper operation.	
Filter Section: All filters are in place and snugly in frames; no bypass, no signs of mold on backside.	
Cooling Coil Section: Coil finned surface clean and free of debris; no indication of carryover, pan clean and draining; biocide tablet in place.	
Supply Fan Section: Fan clean and running smoothly; no belt slippage.	
Heating Section: Area and heat transfer surfaces clean and free of debris.	
Controls: Operating in accordance with sequence of operation; no malfunctions.	
Supply Ductwork: No signs of visible contamination: dust, mold, other debris; no signs of leakage of water in duct.	
Terminal Units: Re-heat and VAV: signs of contamination inside, controls function, signs of water, minimum set-point holding.	
Thermostats: Functioning and calibrated properly.	
Return Air Plenums: Ceiling tiles in place; no signs of contamination above tiles.	
Exhaust Fans: Operating properly; controls functioning.	
HVAC System Standard PM: Refer to vendor's log for any corrections needed or done.	
Cooling Tower Standard PM: Refer to vendor's log for water treatment and any corrections needed or done.	

A maintenance checklist might also be combined with a schedule in one document.
Source: NIOSH/EPA Building Air Quality Handbook. Adapted with permission.

renovation, for example," Fishbeck says, "the building's systems usually aren't designed to circulate enough air to keep those contaminants from affecting patients and staff."

The generic cause of SBS is an elevation of one or more of the following types of contaminants to a potentially harmful level:
- Airborne dust and inorganic particulate matter
- Airborne volatile organic chemicals and vapors
- Allergens, pollens, environmental mold, and bacteria

Individuals affected by SBS might complain of symptoms when working in a particular room or wing of a facility, or complaints might come from workers throughout the building. One characteristic of SBS—an illness that has no defined clinical cause—is that employees' symptoms go away when they leave the facility.

The conditions in a building that contribute to this real or perceived poor indoor air quality (IAQ) are varied and complex, just like the symptoms they cause. People suffering from SBS complain of headaches; eye, nose, and throat irritation; dry cough; dry or itchy skin; dizziness and nausea; difficulty in concentrating; fatigue; and sensitivity to odors.

Causes of SBS

The following elements, which can be exacerbated by humidity or extremes in temperature, are believed to contribute to the poor IAQ that causes SBS:
- *Chemical contaminants from outdoor sources.* Outdoor air that enters a building can become a source of indoor pollution. Vapors from motor vehicle exhaust, plumbing vents, and building exhausts can enter the building through improperly located air-intake vents, windows, and other openings.
- *Chemical contaminants from indoor sources.* Most indoor pollution comes from sources inside the building. Adhesives, upholstery, carpeting, copy machines, manufactured wood products, cleaning agents, and pesticides can emit volatile organic compounds (VOCs), including formaldehyde. At high concentrations, some VOCs can cause chronic, acute health effects—and some are known carcinogens. Tobacco smoke, cleaning and maintenance products, synthetic fragrances in personal care products, and combustion products from stoves can send chemical contaminants into the air.
- *Biological contaminants.* These contaminants—including pollen, bacteria, viruses, and molds—can breed in stagnant water that has accumulated in humidifiers, drain pans, and ducts or on ceiling tiles, insulation, or carpeting. Biological contaminants can cause fever, chills, cough, chest tightness, muscle aches, and allergic reactions.
- *Inadequate ventilation.* Contemporary building energy efficiency has been improved by making buildings more airtight, with less outdoor air ventilation. In many cases, these reduced outdoor ventilation rates make workers uncomfortable and prone to illness.

Preventing SBS

Organizations working to prevent SBS can take one or more of the following steps (in addition to increasing ventilation rates and air distribution):
- *Take special care with special spaces.* Take special care with special areas, such as operating rooms, special procedure rooms, delivery rooms, rooms for patients diagnosed with or suspected of having airborne communicable diseases (for example, pulmonary or laryngeal tuberculosis patients), rooms for patients requiring protective environments (for example, those receiving bone marrow transplants), laboratories, pharmacies, and sterile supply rooms.
- *Monitor how space is used.* If part of a facility built for a specific purpose is later used for a different purpose, the ventilation system might not be appropriate. This point is particularly important in older buildings that have been updated or renovated many times. When you change the way a space is used—for example, using a different type of equipment in a room or on a floor—the HVAC system should be changed to accommodate the new use.
- *Remove or modify pollutants.* Removing or modifying pollutant sources is the most effective way to eliminate a known source of an air-quality problem. Ways to do so include performing routine maintenance of HVAC systems, replacing water-stained ceiling tiles and carpets, venting source emissions to the outdoors, storing paints, solvents, pesticides, and adhesives in closed containers in well-ventilated areas, and allowing time for building materials in new or remodeled areas to off-gas pollutants before occupying those areas.
- *Clean air.* This tactic is a useful supplement to source control and ventilation, but it has limitations. Particle-control devices such as furnace filters are inexpensive but do not capture small particles effectively. High-performance air filters capture small particles but are relatively expensive to install and operate. Absorbent beds might remove some gaseous pollutants, but these devices

can be expensive, and the absorbent material must be replaced often.

- *Ensure that housekeeping is done properly.* If operations, housekeeping, and maintenance tasks are not performed correctly, mold can grow on wet building materials. The housekeeping staff should be instructed to dry spills immediately before mold can accumulate.

- *Check the mechanical system.* A poorly designed mechanical system—or one that has been modified so drastically that it does not meet a building's current requirements—can lead to SBS. A building's systems are designed to maintain the proper balance, filtration, and air pressures; if you are not maintaining the system, it might not be performing up to the original standards for which it was designed. Even if the system is being maintained, organizations might want to have the entire system thoroughly checked and balanced once or twice a year.

- *Wait to occupy a building after construction or renovation.* When new materials are placed in a facility during new construction or renovation, off-gassing of VOCs can occur. Make sure adhesives and paints have time to set before occupying an area. During renovations, check to make sure that renovation activity is not contributing to poor IAQ for those occupying the building.

- *Educate and communicate.* Education and communication are essential for preventive and remedial IAQ–management programs. Key individuals should know the basics of air-quality issues and the facility's plans for handling them. Education on air quality is just as important for administrators and clinical staff as it is for facilities and safety departments. When all employees communicate effectively and understand the causes and consequences of air-quality problems, they can work together to prevent problems from occurring.

Water Distribution Systems and Infection Prevention and Control

Legionella is common in all aquatic environments. Throw in some stagnating water, add a little sediment buildup—of the kind that might result from alterations in plumbing in hospital hot water systems—and you create a perfect opportunity for colonization. Health care organizations report from 600 to 1,300 cases of waterborne *Legionella pneumophila* each year—one of many species of one of many pathogenic biological contaminants.[6] Table 5-3, page 74, lists a number of water-linked outbreaks.

Outbreaks of disease traced to water distribution systems are also caused by opportunistic mold infections, fungi such

as *Aspergillosis* and *Fusariosis,* and bacteria—some of which can replicate in relatively pure water—such as *Pseudomonas aeruginosa, Stenotrophomonas maltophilia,* and various mycobacterial species. Annual mortality from waterborne *P aeruginosa nosocomial pneumonia* might be as high as 1,400.[7]

Preventing Pathogens from Colonizing

The key to preventing such pathogens from colonizing in water-based utility systems is to ensure that equipment that recirculates water continuously is properly designed, accurately installed, and adequately maintained. Specifically, pathogenic biological agents must be managed in cooling towers, domestic hot water systems, and aerosolizing water systems, including showers, humidifiers, and fountains.

As with airborne contaminants, organizations should perform a risk assessment to identify areas serving the individuals most susceptible to waterborne contaminants as well. (Actually, one assessment process can be used for both kinds of contaminants.) Red flags would include dead ends in the plumbing system or portions that have been shut off for any reason, as they are most likely to hold stagnant water.

Finding Contaminants

Where in water distribution systems are contaminants found? Where are they not? The following spots have all been known to harbor waterborne nosocomial pathogens in health care facilities[8]:

- *Sinks.* These are not considered an important factor, but if there is reason to think that a sink might be implicated in the spread of gram-negative bacteria, which can last in wet environments for a long time, staff should not use it to wash their hands. (This is why routine daily cleaning is so important.)

- *Faucet aerators and handheld shower heads.* Experts do not know how often aerators are the source of infection but say there is no need to remove all aerators and screens or to disinfect them.

- *Ice and ice machines.* Because there is no microbial standard for these, routine cultures are not recommended, but the CDC guidelines include a regular program of disinfection of ice machines.

- *Eyewash stations.* Because source water for these infrequently used facilities might stand in incoming pipes at room temperature for months or years, the American National Standards Institute (ANSI) recommends that eyewash stations should nonetheless be flushed weekly.

- *Dental-unit water systems.* Clean-water units should be disinfected weekly.

- *Water baths.* Organizations should develop policies for routine cleaning, disinfection, and changing of water (to which a germicide has been added) in baths used to thaw fresh plasma or cryoprecipitate or to warm bottles of peritoneal dialysate before use. Or, eliminate the problem by using warm-air cabinets or a microwave.
- *Tubs.* Whether used in physical therapy, burn wound cleaning, or bathing babies, tubs should be subject to strict disinfection protocols between patients.
- *Toilets.* There is no need to pour disinfectants into the bowl. Cleaning with a scouring powder and brush is sufficient. Keep surfaces clean with a disinfection solution.
- *Dialysis water.* The CDC suggests that organizations sample both the water used to prepare dialysis fluid (whether distilled, deionized, reverse-osmosis, or softened) and the dialysate itself monthly; the water should have less than 200 bacteria/mL, the dialysate less than 2,000 bacteria/mL.

Flowers might help support the patient's well-being, but cannot be in the rooms of immunocompromised patients. For rooms that can receive flowers, staff—ideally support personnel with no patient contact—should use gloves and wash hands after handling flowers; vase water should be changed at least every other day and disposed of into sinks not used for hand washing, and the vases themselves cleaned and disinfected after use.

One of the most frequently overlooked sources of contaminants is tap water if used to rinse semicritical equipment (such as tracheal suction tubing), to irrigate during colonoscopy, or to rinse burn patients.[6] Patients are also exposed when they shower, bathe, drink, or gargle water in the hospital.

Experts suggest using sterile water for immunocompromised patients or disposable sterile sponges instead of showering, using only sterile water in large-volume room air humidifiers that

Table 5-3: Hospital Water–Linked Outbreaks

Microorganisms	Reservoir	Infection
P. paucimobilis	Water bottles for rising tracheal suction	Pneumonia
S. marcescens	Water of humidifiers	Pneumonia
M. xenopi	Hot water taps	Pneumonia
M. chelonei	Contaminated equipment	Otitis
M. chelonei	Contaminated water tank	Nasal septum cellulites
L. pneumophila	Hospital water, cooling towers	Pneumonia
Acinetobacter species	Water bath used to thaw fresh plasma	Bacteremia
P. aeruginosa	Water bath used to thaw cryoprecipitate	Bacteremia
P. aeruginosa	Tub water contamination	Folliculitis, skin infections
C. difficile	Bath	Diarrhea

This list is representative rather than exhaustive.

Source: Rangel-Fraustro M.S.: Water. In Wenzel R.P., Brewer T.F., Butzler J.P. (eds.): A Guide to Infection Control in the Hospital, 2nd ed. International Society for Infectious Diseases; 2002. http://www.isid.org/publications/guide_infection_contr.shtml. Used with permission.

create aerosols (and only if they can be sterilized or subjected to high-level disinfection at least daily), replacing water-containing devices with those not requiring water to work, and keeping water circulating at temperatures below 20°C or above 60°C. Where water cannot be eliminated, it should be disinfected with chemicals or heat and regularly monitored.[9]

Note that disinfection can be done continuously or on an as-needed basis. Focal disinfection methods (for example, ultraviolet light) are applied at a specific point in a water distribution system, and water is disinfected as it passes that point; these are easy to install but ineffective against systemwide contamination. On the other hand, systemic disinfectants such as chlorine dioxide or copper-silver ions can be effective even at the farthest taps, but they must be able to penetrate or remove biofilm, which protects valves, fittings, and pipe walls from chemical disinfectants.

Best of all, of course, is to avoid the buildup of biofilm and the corrosion of distribution lines and tank surfaces that cause poor water quality in the first place and are themselves caused by aging systems or design flaws.

As a preventive measure, the AIA in 2001 recommended raising tap-water temperatures from 105°F to 120°F in hospitals. (The CDC recommendation is for 124°F and includes a scalding risk assessment.) Facilities can store water at higher temperatures as long as mixing valves reduce the temperature at the tap to within the recommended range.[9]

Legionella

Legionellosis is an infectious disease caused by bacteria belonging to the genus *Legionella*. *Legionella* is a primary target of IC in utility systems and for good reason. It thrives on scale and biofilm, loves stagnant water, and prefers temperatures between 80°F and 120°F. Legionnaires' disease infects between 8,000 and 18,000 Americans each year and can cause death in up to 5% to 30% of cases, according to the CDC.[10]

At the highest risk are people with HIV, organ transplant recipients, people who are immunocompromised because of illness or chemotherapy, smokers, people over age 65, and people with respiratory illnesses. Most cases go undetected because U.S. hospitals do not routinely use special lab tests required for diagnosis and because many physicians treat pneumonia without seeking an underlying cause.[11] At the same time, most cases can be treated successfully with antibiotics, and healthy people typically recover from infection.[10]

Legionnaires' disease can have symptoms like many other forms of pneumonia, so it can be hard to diagnose at first. Signs of the disease can include a high fever, chills, and a cough. Some people may also suffer from muscle aches and headaches. Chest x-rays are needed to find the pneumonia caused by the bacteria, and other tests can be done on sputum (phlegm), as well as on blood or urine, to find evidence of the bacteria in the body. The symptoms usually begin 2 to 14 days after being exposed to the bacteria.[12] Figure 5-2 on page 76 presents a list of issues every clinician should know about Legionnaires' disease.

CDC Recommendations

The CDC recommends that organizations establish a surveillance process to detect health care-associated Legionnaires' disease, including performing laboratory diagnostic tests on suspected cases, especially in at-risk patients. Whenever laboratory tests confirm a case of Legionnaires' disease, or whenever two or more suspected cases occur during a six-month period, an organization should conduct an epidemiologic investigation to look for previously unidentified cases and should begin intensive prospective surveillance for additional cases. An organization that treats severely immunocompromised patients should also implement culture strategies and potable water and fixture treatment measures, as outlined in the CDC's *Guidelines for Environmental Infection Control in Health Care Facilities*.[12]

An outbreak, which the CDC defines as continued health care-associated transmission, should trigger an environmental assessment to determine the source of *Legionella* species, including collecting water samples from potential aerosolized water sources and promptly instituting system decontamination measures when a source is identified. Hyperchlorination and superheating the water are two one-time decontamination methods used; another is the use of chlorine dioxide, which the CDC considers an unresolved issue.

According to the International Society for Infectious Diseases, follow-up cultures should be done at two-week intervals for three months after an incident to evaluate the actions taken. If no further positive cultures are found, collect monthly cultures for another three months; if positive cultures are found, reassess and modify the implemented control measures, implement decontamination again, and consider combination methods to decontaminate the water.[13]

Figure 5-2: What Every Clinician Needs to Know About Legionnaires' Disease

- Who should be tested for Legionnaires' disease?
  - Hospitalized patients with enigmatic pneumonia
  - Patients with enigmatic pneumonia sufficiently severe to require care in the intensive care unit
  - Compromised host with pneumonia
  - Patients with pneumonia in the setting of a Legionellosis outbreak
  - Patients who fail to respond to treatment with a ß-lactam or cephalosporin
  - Patients with a travel history (patients that have traveled away from their home within two weeks before the onset of illness)
  - Patients suspected of nosocomial pneumonia with unknown etiology

- **How do I test for Legionnaires' disease?**
  - Urinary antigen assay and culture of respiratory secretions on selective media are the preferred diagnostic tests for Legionnaires' disease.
  - Sensitivity and specificity of diagnostic tests

- **Why is it important to obtain a respiratory specimen for culture of possible Legionella infection?**

  Isolation of Legionella from respiratory secretions, lung tissue, pleural fluid, or a normally sterile site is still an important method for diagnosis, despite the convenience and specificity of urinary antigen testing. Investigations of outbreaks of Legionnaires' disease rely on both clinical and environmental isolates. Clinical and environmental isolates can be compared using monoclonal antibody and molecular techniques. Because Legionella are commonly found in the environment, clinical isolates are necessary to interpret the findings of an environmental investigation.

- **What is the preferred treatment for Legionnaires' disease?**
  - If your patient has Legionnaires' disease, please see the most recent guidelines from the Infectious Diseases Society of America (IDSA) for community-acquired pneumonia.
  - For patients with Pontiac fever: It is a self-limited illness that does not benefit from antibiotic treatment. Complete recovery usually occurs within one week.

- **Why do I need to ask patients about travel in the 14 days before onset of disease?**

  Although outbreaks of travel-associated Legionellosis are infrequently identified, more than 20% of all cases are thought to be associated with recent travel. Outbreaks of Legionnaires' disease among travelers are difficult to detect because of the low attack rate, long incubation period, and the dispersal of persons from the source of the outbreak. Timely reporting of travel-associated cases could allow early identification and control of known sources of infection.

- **How common is Legionnaires' disease?**

  Each year an estimated 8,000 to 18,000 hospitalized cases occur in the United States. However, accurate data reflecting the true incidence of disease are not available because of underutilization of diagnostic testing and under-reporting. It is a common cause of severe pneumonia requiring hospitalization. The majority of reported cases are sporadic. Travel-associated outbreaks, outbreaks in community settings, and nosocomial and occupational outbreaks are common.

- **Where does Legionella come from?**

  Legionella can be found in natural, freshwater environments, but it is present in insufficient numbers to cause disease. Potable (drinking) water systems, whirlpool spas, and cooling towers provide the three conditions needed for Legionella transmission: heat, stasis, and aerosolization; therefore, these are common sources of outbreaks.

- **What are epidemiologic risk factors for Legionellosis?**
  - Recent travel with an overnight stay outside of the home
  - Exposure to whirlpool spas
  - Recent repairs or maintenance work on domestic plumbing
  - Renal or hepatic failure
  - Diabetes
  - Systemic malignancy
  - Smoking
  - Immune system disorders

- **How should you report Legionellosis?**

  Legionellosis is a nationally notifiable disease. Report cases of Legionellosis to your local or state health department. Call, fax, or mail this information to your local or state health department within seven days of diagnosis. Prompt reporting could allow early identification and control of known sources of infection.[10]

(continued on next page)

Figure 5-2: *continued*

– LEGIONELLOSIS CASE REPORT –

Patient's Name: _____ Hospital: _____
(Last, First, M.I.)   (Telephone No.)

Address: _____ Patient Chart No.: _____
(Number, Street, Apt. No., City, State)   (Zip Code)

-- Patient identifier information is not transmitted to CDC --

DEPARTMENT OF HEALTH & HUMAN SERVICES
Centers for Disease Control
and Prevention (CDC)
Atlanta, Georgia 30333

LEGIONELLOSIS CASE REPORT
(DISEASE CAUSED BY ANY LEGIONELLA SPECIES)

Form Approved OMB No. 0920-0009

– PATIENT INFORMATION –

1. State Health Dept. Case No.
2. Reporting State:
3. (CDC Use Only) Case No.
4. County of Residence
5. State of Residence
6. Occupation:

7a. Date of Birth: Mo. Day Year
7b. Age: 1 Days 2 Mos. 3 Years
8. Sex: 1 Male 2 Female
9. Ethnicity: 1 Hispanic/Latino 2 Not Hispanic/Latino 9 Unk
10. Race: 1 American Indian/Alaskan Native 2 Asian 3 Black or African American 4 Native Hawaiian or Other Pacific Islander 5 White 9 Unk

11. Possible sources of exposure:

IN THE TWO WEEKS BEFORE ONSET, DID PATIENT:

a) Travel or stay overnight somewhere other than usual residence? CITY   LODGING

1 Yes 2 No 9 Unk   If **Yes**, give cities and lodging where available: _____

* For suspected travel related cases, please contact CDC or pertinent state health departments immediately.

b) Have dental work? 1 Yes 2 No 9 Unk If **Yes**, name of dental office: _____

c) Visit a hospital as an outpatient? 1 Yes 2 No 9 Unk If **Yes**, name of hospital: _____

d) Work in a hospital? 1 Yes 2 No 9 Unk If **Yes**, name of hospital: _____

12. Was case hospital related (nosocomial)?

2 Not nosocomial: No inpatient or outpatient hospital visits in the 10 days prior to onset of symptoms.
3 Possibly nosocomial: Patient hospitalized 2 - 9 days before onset of legionella infection.
9 Unk
1 Definitely nosocomial: Patient hospitalized continuously for ≥ 10 days before onset of legionella infection.
8 Other(Specify) _____

13. Was this patient's legionella infection: (check one)

1 Associated with outbreak (Specify location): _____
2 Sporadic case 9 Unk

– CLINICAL ILLNESS –

14. Diagnosis: (check one)

1 Legionnaires' Disease (Pneumonia, X-ray diagnosed) 8 Other (Specify) _____
2 Pontiac fever (fever, myalgia without pneumonia) 9 Unk

15. Date of symptom onset of Legionellosis Mo. Day Year
16. Was patient hospitalized for Legionellosis? 1 Yes 2 No 9 Unk Hospital name: _____ Hospital address: _____
17. Outcome of illness: 1 Survived 9 Unk 2 Died

– CASE DEFINITION –

Confirmed case has a compatible clinical history and meets at least one of the following criteria:

1) isolation of *Legionella* species from lung tissue, respiratory secretions, pleural fluid, blood or other sterile site
2) demonstration of *L. pneumophila*, serogroup 1, in lung tissue, respiratory secretions, or pleural fluid by direct fluorescent antibody testing
3) fourfold or greater rise in immunoflourescent antibody titer to *L. pneumophila*, serogroup 1, to 128 or greater
4) detection of *L. pneumophila* serogroup 1 antigen in urine

Public reporting burden of this collection of information is estimated to average 20 minutes per response, including the time for reviewing instructions, searching existing data sources, gathering and maintaining the data needed, and completing and reviewing the collection of information. An agency may not conduct or sponsor, and a person is not required to respond to a collection of information unless it displays a currently valid OMB control number. Send comments regarding this burden estimate or any other aspect of this collection of information, including suggestions for reducing this burden to CDC, Project Clearance Officer, 1600 Clifton Road, MS D-74, Atlanta, GA 30333, ATTN: PRA (0920-0009). Do not send the completed form to this address. While your response is voluntary your cooperation is necessary for the understanding and control of this disease.

CDC 52.56 Rev. 02/2003   – LEGIONELLOSIS CASE REPORT –   Page 1 of 2

(continued on next page)

Figure 5-2: *continued*

– LEGIONELLOSIS CASE REPORT –

– METHOD OF DIAGNOSIS –

PLEASE CHECK ALL METHODS OF DIAGNOSIS WHICH APPLY

1☐ **Culture Positive: If Yes,**
Date:
Mo.   Day   Year

Site: 1☐ lung biopsy   2☐ respiratory secretions   3☐ pleural fluid   4☐ blood   8☐ Other: (Specify) _____

Species: _____   **Serogroup:** _____

2☐ **DFA Positive: If Yes,**
Date:
Mo.   Day   Year

Site: 1☐ lung biopsy   2☐ respiratory secretions   3☐ pleural fluid   4☐ blood   8☐ Other: (Specify) _____

Species: _____   **Serogroup:** _____

3☐ **Fourfold rise in antibody titer: If Yes,**
Date:
Mo.   Day   Year   List Species and Serogroup in assay used:

Initial (acute) titer 1: _____   **Species:** _____   **Serogroup:** _____

Convalescent titer 1: _____   **Species:** _____   **Serogroup:** _____

4☐ **Urine Antigen Positive: If Yes,**
Date:
Mo.   Day   Year

– INTERVIEWER IDENTIFICATION –

Interviewer's Name:
_____

Affiliation:
_____

Telephone No.:
__ __ __ - __ __ __ - __ __ __ __

Date of Interview:
Mo.   Day   Year

– CDC USE ONLY –

Local Health Dept. Please submit this document to:
State/DHD/SSS via your CD reporting clerk

State Health Dept. Return completed form to:
Respiratory Diseases Branch, Mailstop C23
National Center for Infectious Diseases
Centers for Disease Control and Prevention
1600 Clifton Rd. NE
Atlanta, GA 30333

Check the appropriate answer: Serogroup: _____

1☐ *L. pneumophila*   6☐ *L. feeleii*

2☐ *L. bozemanii*   7☐ *L. longbeachae*

3☐ *L. dumoffii*   8☐ Mixed: (specify)_____

4☐ *L. gormanii*   88☐ Other: (specify)_____

5☐ *L. micdadei*   99☐ Unk

– COMMENTS –

_____

_____

_____

_____

_____

_____

Prevention Methods

Stopping *Legionella* before it infects patients, staff, or visitors is the crux of the matter. Visual inspection and periodic maintenance of the system are the best ways to control growth of *Legionella* and related organisms, according to the Occupational Safety and Health Administration (OSHA).

Toward this end, cooling towers should be located so that their drift is directed away from air intakes. Experts suggest that twice-yearly cleaning and disinfecting, normally prior to seasonal start-up and shutdown, should include drift eliminators, which are essential for all towers, and regular maintenance should include the addition of an appropriate biocide such as bromine or chlorine. High concentrations of organic matter and dissolved solids in the water will reduce the effectiveness of any biocidal agent; for this reason, each pump should be equipped with a "bleed," and make-up water should be supplied to reduce the concentration of dissolved solids. Decorative fountains should likewise be kept clean and should undergo regular chemical treatment to control microbiological growth.

In addition to delivering water to outlets at higher temperatures, organizations can take other measures. Consider recirculation of the water in the system, make sure any dead ends are short, and use self-draining water pipes between valve and shower. The hot water tank, which when large often contains cool zones near the base where scale and sediment accumulate, should be drained periodically and cleaned with chlorine solution, if possible, followed by thorough rinsing. (The Maryland Department of Health and Mental Hygiene recommends that instantaneous or semi-instantaneous water heaters should be used instead of tanks.) Domestic hot-water recirculation pumps should run continuously and be excluded from energy conservation measures.[14]

OSHA Recommendations

OSHA has identified the following alternative means to control *Legionella* growth:

- The use of metal ions such as copper or silver, which have a biocidal effect, in solution
- Ozonization
- Ultraviolet radiation on incoming water lines or recirculating systems

The Joint Commission does not require organizations to regularly culture their water systems for *Legionella*, but a local authority having jurisdiction might do so. The issue of routine sampling inspires heated debate. The CDC recommends maintaining a high index of suspicion for *Legionella* as a clinical diagnosis but culturing only after diagnosis in hospitals that do not serve at-risk patients who require a protective environment. *Legionella*, the agency points out, is indigenous to the water: If you culture for it, you will find it and then have to take action, even though not all occurrences will lead to disease.

Likewise, OSHA advises analyzing samples only from a source suspected of being contaminated. On the other hand, the Maryland Department of Health and Mental Hygiene recommends that acute care hospitals in the state routinely sample plumbing systems for *Legionella*,[15] and the Allegheny County (Pennsylvania) Health Department says once a year is sufficient.[16] According to the Maryland guidelines, risk factors occurring at each facility, including the following, should dictate the time schedule for such assessment[13]:

- Engineering, age, and complexity of the facility's hot water system
- Facility's remediation history and frequency
- Patient mix and the number of transplant, chemotherapy, and other immunocompromised patients served in the facility
- Prior Legionnaires' history

What are facility managers to do? Consult with the organization's IC professional; review the facts, including the following; and make an informed decision:

- Surveys involving 264 hospitals in the United States, the United Kingdom, and Canada showed that nearly half of facilities found no *Legionella* in domestic water systems.
- OSHA and others have tables listing appropriate responses to various *Legionella* counts in buildings occupied by healthy people, but there is no specific guidance available for risk zones.
- Sampling cannot replace preventive maintenance or testing of patients with pneumonia.
- If you do not implement preventive and corrective measures, sampling might hurt your defense in lawsuits.
- Sampling can be an impetus for risk reduction and should increase communication between facility management, IC, and the medical staff.

In any event, all sampling should follow organizational policy, which should be developed in close collaboration with IC professionals and approved by both the administration and the IC committee.

References

1. Beaver M.: Air and waterborne pathogens are resilient. *Infection Control Today,* Apr. 16, 2008. http://www.infectioncontroltoday.com/articles/airborne-andwaterborne-pathogens.html (accessed Jun. 3, 2009).

2. National Institute for Occupational Safety and Health: NIOSH-Funded Study Simulates Hospital Room to Test UV System for Employee TB Protection. Apr. 29, 2003. http://www.cdc.gov/niosh/updates/uvsysfortb.html (accessed Jun. 3, 2009).

3. Streifel A.J.: Health-care IAQ: Guidance for infection control. *Air Conditioning and Refrigeration Journal,* Apr.–Jun. 2001. http://www.ishrae.in/journals/2001apr/article04.html (accessed Jun. 3, 2009).

4. Cox R.: *Effective Design of Heating, Ventilation and Air-conditioning Systems for Healthcare Facilities.* World Market Series: Business Briefings. http://www.bbriefings.com/pdf/747/ACFCFF.pdf (accessed Jun. 3, 2009).

5. Aerobiological Engineering. The Pennsylvania State University Graduate School of Architectural Engineering. http://www.engr.psu.edu/ae/iec/abe/index.asp (accessed Jun. 3, 2009).

6. Burns S.: Water: Is it a breeding ground for bacteria in your facility? *Infection Control Today,* Oct. 1, 2002. http://www.infectioncontroltoday.com/articles/2a1feat2.html (accessed Jun. 5, 2009).

7. Jurasek G.: Danger on tap in hospitals. *Pulmonary Reviews.Com* 7(9), Sept. 2002. http://www.pulmonaryreviews.com/sep02/pr_sep02_tap.html (accessed Jun. 5, 2009).

8. Ulrich R.S., et al.: Healthcare Leadership: A Review of the Research Literature on Evidence-Based Healthcare Design, 2008. http://www/healthdesign.org/hcleader/HCLeader_5_LitReviewWP.pdf (accessed May 31, 2009).

9. American Institute of Architects: *Guidelines for Design and Construction of Hospital and Health Care Facilities, 2001.*Washington: Jun. 2001.

10. Centers for Disease Control and Prevention: *Legionellosis Resource Site.* Aug. 18, 2008. http://www.cdc.gov/legionella/index.htm (accessed Jun. 5, 2009).

11. Wenzel R.P., Brewer T.F., Butzler J.P. (eds.): *A Guide to Infection Control in the Hospital,* 2nd ed. Boston, MA: International Society for Infectious Diseases, 2002. http://www.isid.org/publications/guide_infection_contr.shtml (accessed Jun. 3, 2009).

12. Occupational Safety & Health Administration: *OSHA Technical Manual. Section III, Chapter 7: Legionnaire's Disease.* http://www.osha.gov/dts/osta/otm/otm_iii/otm_iii_7.html (accessed Jun. 5, 2009).

13. Maryland Department of Health and Mental Hygiene: *Report of the Maryland Scientific Working Group to Study Legionella in Water Systems in Healthcare Institutions.* Jun. 14, 2000. http://www.dhmh.state.md.us/html/legionella.htm (accessed Jun. 5, 2009).

14. Allegheny County Health Department: *Approaches to Prevention and Control of Legionella Infection in Allegheny County Health Care Facilities,* 1st revised ed. Jan. 1997. http://www.legionella.org/achd_guideline.pdf (accessed Feb. 5, 2009).

15. Joint Commission Resources (JCR): *Care Delivery and the Environment of Care: A Teamwork Approach.* Oakbrook Terrace, IL: JCR, 2003.

16. Freije M.R.: Testing the waters: Facts to consider when deciding whether to sample for *Legionella. Health Facil Manage* 15, May 2003. http://www.hfmmagazine.com/hfmmagazine_app/jsp/articledisplay.jsp?dcrpath=HFMMAGAZINE/PubsNewsArticleGen/data/Backup/0406HFM_DEPT_Codes (accessed Jun. 5, 2009).

Chapter 6

Construction and Renovation

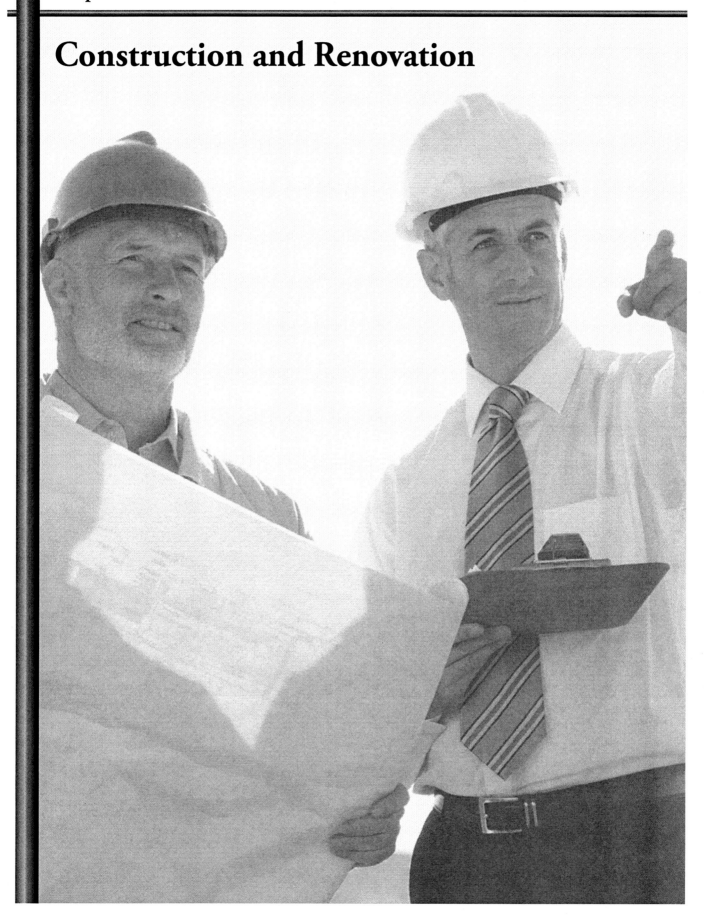

Construction and Renovation

Construction and renovation pose many threats for contracting health care–associated infections (HAIs) and continue to cause concerns in health care facilities. One factor of concern is the mounting understanding of various illnesses and the compromised immune systems that have become characteristics of hospitalized individuals as more care is delivered on an outpatient basis. Another factor is the increased volume of new construction being undertaken. By 2007, approximately $44 billion in hospital construction—including new facilities, renovation, and expansion—was in the design stage.[1] Couple that with the fact that an estimated 5,000 deaths are associated with construction-related HAIs each year,[2] and that sick patients are more vulnerable to disease and infection than the general population,[1] the collision of construction and infection emerges as an added challenge for an infection preventionist.

Dispersal of airborne or waterborne microorganisms during construction activities has been linked to a variety of environmental factors that cause the spread of HAIs. This chapter explores the risk assessment process of infection prevention and control (IC) through IC guidelines and recommendations. It emphasizes the importance of preparation practices before construction begins, as well as safety measures taken during and after these types of projects. While outlining responsibilities in the process, the chapter also considers the role of architectural design in preventing and controlling infection in the health care setting.

Infection Prevention and Control Risk Assessment

HAIs have been linked to environmental factors, such as new fireproofing insulation, carpeting, and ventilation system humidifiers, among many other factors. For this reason, The Joint Commission addresses IC in the Environment of Care (EC) standards by requiring organizations to manage the environment during demolition, renovation, or new construction events to reduce any risk to those within the organization. The standards also require an organization to measure its performance using state rules and regulations;

the *Guidelines for the Design and Construction of Hospitals and Health Care Facilities*, 2001 Edition, published by the American Institute of Architects (AIA) or its updated version; or other reputable standards and guidelines of equivalence.

The health care organization should also conduct a preconstruction risk assessment for air quality requirements, IC, utility requirements, noise, vibration, and other hazards that can affect the care, treatment, and services provided and should take actions, as needed, based on its assessment of the environment.

The AIA guidelines referenced in the standards have evolved to include engineering systems, IC, and safety, as well as architectural guidelines, and are intended to serve as minimum construction requirements. Along with The Joint Commission, authorities in 42 states and several federal agencies use the AIA guidelines as a reference, code, or standard when reviewing construction designs and plans and completing health care facilities.

The American Institute of Architecture Guidelines

The AIA's guidelines include an expansion of the EC chapter by emphasizing detailed functional program requirements. This edition also contains material on infection control risk assessments (ICRAs), IC risk mitigation recommendations, and a chapter focusing on common requirements for all health care facility types. Its section on hospitals includes the following[3]:

- Single-bed rooms as the minimum standard for medical/surgical and postpartum nursing units in general hospitals
- Bed clearances and bedside documentation areas in critical care units
- Sections on intermediate care units in general hospitals, observation units in emergency departments, freestanding emergency facilities, and in-hospital skilled nursing units
- Content on decontamination areas and appendix language on surge capacity in emergency departments
- A section on in-hospital psychiatric nursing units
- A chapter on small inpatient primary care hospitals

The Centers for Disease Control and Prevention Recommendations

Organizations planning to tear down, build up, or alter facilities will also want to consult the American Society for Healthcare Engineering (ASHE) Infection Control Risk Assessment for construction and the Centers for Disease Control and Prevention (CDC) 2003 Guidelines for Environmental Infection Control in Health Care Facilities.[4] Sidebar 6-1 on pages 85–86 outlines CDC guidelines on construction, renovation, remediation, and demolition.

Reducing Risk in Architecture

Poor air quality and ventilation combined with having two or more patients in the same room are prime causes of infections.[5] For reasons such as this, the interior design aspect of construction and renovation projects is important in IC.

Including infection preventionists in facility design from the very earliest stages can go a long way to protect patients, clients, or residents. For example, these professionals should play a substantial role in determining the appropriate location of negative-airflow rooms in areas where high-risk patients will be treated (for example, emergency department, recovery room, bronchoscopy suite). Although fashion or convenience might dictate otherwise, the infection preventionist will insist on using common sense and science as a guide.

AIA Recommendations

An important and controversial design issue involves placing sinks inside the patient room or inside the patient's toilet room. The AIA guidelines call for both, with the former situated near the exit and outside any privacy curtain. They weigh in on another debate by stating clearly that a "hand-washing facility" means a sink with running water, as opposed to a dispenser of waterless agents.

Another important design issue is carpets in health care facilities, as carpet should always have impermeable backing, chemically welded seams, and antistatic properties. Easy cleaning is key, as some of the newer carpeting materials are very thin rather than plush and have vinyl backings. Liquids stay on top of the material and can be easily cleaned.

The life cycle of carpet is another factor in the carpet versus no-carpet issue. How well will the carpet stand up to frequent cleaning and decontamination? Carpets should be vacuumed daily and periodically steam cleaned. How much will it cost to maintain it? And what will you do with patients, clients, or residents while carpets are being decontaminated?

Carpeting should definitely be avoided in high-risk areas because the cleaning process itself might aerosolize fungal spores.

Floor surfaces that should be easy to clean without hazardous chemicals are a concern. The AIA guidelines for design of neonatal intensive care units (NICUs) cites medical-grade sheet flooring, and it is here in the NICU that AIA requirements are most stringent. Health care organizations determined to make IC a top priority might want to consider adapting AIA's NICU guidelines for general use. In addition to medical-grade sheet flooring, these guidelines specify ceiling finishes be made so that particles can't pass from the cavity above the ceiling plane into the patient area.

Sidebar 6-2 on page 87 offers a list of resources for regulatory or professional guidelines regarding construction and IC. In addition, the Facility Guidelines Institute will update the AIA guidelines. The new guidelines will be available in January 2010.

Before Construction

The point of the assessment is to identify and mitigate the effects of construction activities on air quality and heating, ventilation, air conditioning (HVAC) systems; water supply and plumbing; utility requirements; and other factors that affect IC including construction staging and work methods.

As outlined in the AIA guidelines, the assessment before construction must address, at a minimum, the following elements[3]:

- Impact of disruption on patients and employees
- Patient placement or relocation
- Placement of effective barriers to protect susceptible patients from airborne contaminants such as *Aspergillus* species
- Air handling needs in surgical services, airborne infection isolation (AII) and protective environment (PE) rooms, laboratories, local exhaust systems for hazardous agents, and other special areas
- Determination of additional numbers of AII or PE rooms
- Consideration of the domestic water system to limit *Legionella* species and other waterborne opportunistic pathogens
- Assessment of internal and external construction projects to include patient protection from demolition, ventilation, water management following planned or unplanned power outages, movement of debris, traffic flow, cleanup, and certification

Sidebar 6-1: Centers for Disease Control and Prevention Guidelines on Construction, Renovation, Remediation, Repair, and Demolition

- Establish a multidisciplinary team that includes an infection preventionist to coordinate demolition, construction, and renovation projects, and consider proactive preventive measures at the inception. Create and maintain summary statements of the team's activities.

- Educate the construction team and health care staff in immunocompromised patient care areas regarding the airborne infection risks associated with construction projects, dispersal of fungal spores during such activities, and methods to control the dissemination of fungal spores.

- Incorporate mandatory adherence agreements for infection prevention and control (IC) into construction contracts, with penalties for noncompliance and mechanisms to ensure timely correction of problems.

- Establish and maintain surveillance for airborne environmental diseases (such as *Aspergillus* species), as appropriate, during construction, renovation, repair, and demolition activities to ensure the health and safety of immunocompromised patients by doing the following:
  - Use active surveillance to monitor for airborne infections in immunocompromised patients.
  - Periodically review the facility's microbiologic, histopathologic, and postmortem data to identify additional cases.
  - If cases of *Aspergillus* species or other health care–associated airborne fungal infections occur, aggressively pursue the diagnosis with tissue biopsies and cultures, as feasible.

- Implement IC measures relevant to construction, renovation, maintenance, demolition, and repair.
  - Before the project gets under way, perform the following IC risk assessment to define the scope of the activity and the need for barrier measures:
    - Determine if immunocompromised patients may be at risk for exposure to fungal spores from dust generated during the project.
    - Develop a contingency plan to prevent such exposures.
  - Implement the following IC measures for external demolition and construction activities:
    - Determine if the facility can operate temporarily on recirculated air; if feasible, seal off adjacent air intakes.
    - If this is not possible or practical, check the low-efficiency (roughing) filter banks frequently and replace as needed to avoid buildup of particulates.
    - Seal windows and reduce, wherever possible, other sources of outside air intrusion (such as open doors in stairwells and corridors), particularly in protective environment areas.

- Avoid damaging the underground water system (such as buried pipes) to prevent soil and dust contamination of the water.
  - Implement the following IC measures for internal construction activities:
    - Construct barriers to prevent dust from construction areas from entering patient care areas; ensure that barriers are impermeable to fungal spores and in compliance with local fire codes.
    - Seal off and block return air vents if rigid barriers are used for containment.
    - Implement dust control measures on surfaces and divert pedestrian traffic away from work zones.
    - Relocate patients whose rooms are adjacent to work zones, depending on their immune status, the scope of the project, the potential for generation of dust or water aerosols, and the methods used to control these aerosols.

- Perform those engineering and work site–related IC measures, as needed, for internal construction, repairs, and renovations by doing the following:
  - Ensure proper operation of the air handling system in the affected area after erection of barriers and before the room or area is set to negative pressure.
  - Create and maintain negative air pressure in work zones adjacent to patient care areas and ensure that required engineering controls are maintained.
  - Monitor negative airflow inside rigid barriers.
  - Monitor barriers and ensure integrity of the construction barriers; repair gaps or breaks in barrier joints.
  - Seal windows in work zones if practical; use window chutes for disposal of large pieces of debris as needed, but ensure that the negative pressure differential for the area is maintained.
  - Direct pedestrian traffic from construction zones away from patient care areas to minimize dispersion of dust.
  - Provide construction crews with (1) designated entrances, corridors, and elevators wherever practical; (2) essential services (such as toilet facilities) and convenience services (such as vending machines);

(continued on next page)

Sidebar 6-1: *continued*

(3) protective clothing (such as coveralls, footgear, and headgear) for travel to patient care areas; and (4) a space or anteroom for changing clothing and storing equipment.

– Clean work zones and their entrances daily by (1) wet-wiping tools and tool carts before their removal from the work zone; (2) placing mats with tacky surfaces inside the entrance; and (3) covering debris and securing this covering before removing debris from the work zone.

– In patient care areas, for major repairs that include removal of ceiling tiles and disruption of the space above the false ceiling, use plastic sheets or prefabricated plastic units to contain dust; use a negative pressure system within this enclosure to remove dust; and either pass air through an industrial-grade, portable high-efficiency particulate air (HEPA) filter capable of filtration rates of 300–800 ft/min or exhaust air directly to the outside.

– Upon completion of the project, clean the work zone according to facility procedures and install barrier curtains to contain dust and debris before removing rigid barriers.

– Flush the water system to clear sediment from pipes to minimize waterborne microorganism proliferation.

– Restore appropriate air changes per hour (ACH), humidity, and pressure differential; clean or replace air filters; dispose of spent filters.

• Use airborne particle sampling as a tool to evaluate barrier integrity.

• Commission the heating, ventilation, and air conditioning (HVAC) system for newly constructed health care facilities and renovated spaces before occupancy and use, with emphasis on ensuring proper ventilation for operating rooms, airborne infection isolation rooms, and protective environment (PE) areas.

• If a case of health care-associated *Aspergillus* species or other opportunistic environmental airborne fungal disease occurs during or immediately after construction, implement appropriate follow-up measures:

  ○ Review pressure differential monitoring documentation to verify that pressure differentials in the construction zone and in PE rooms are appropriate for their settings.

  ○ Implement corrective engineering measures to restore proper pressure differentials as needed.

  ○ Conduct a prospective search for additional cases and intensify retrospective epidemiologic review of the hospital's medical and laboratory records.

  ○ If no epidemiologic evidence of ongoing transmission exists, continue routine maintenance in the area to prevent health care-acquired fungal disease.

• If no epidemiologic evidence exists of ongoing transmission of fungal disease, conduct the following environmental assessment to find and eliminate the source:

  ○ Collect environmental samples from potential sources of airborne fungal spores, preferably by using a high-volume air sampler rather than settle plates.

  ○ If either an environmental source of airborne fungi or an engineering problem with filtration or pressure differentials is identified, promptly perform corrective measures to eliminate the source and route of entry.

  ○ Use an Environmental Protection Agency–registered antifungal biocide (such as copper-8-quinolinolate) for decontaminating structural materials.

  ○ If an environmental source of airborne fungi is not identified, review infection prevention and control measures, including engineering controls, to identify potential areas for correction or improvement.

  ○ If possible, perform molecular subtyping of *Aspergillus* species isolated from patients and the environment to compare their strain identities.

• If air-supply systems to high-risk areas (such as PE rooms) are not optimal, use portable, industrial-grade HEPA filters on a temporary basis until rooms with optimal air-handling systems become available.

Source: Schulster L., Chinn R.Y.W.: Guidelines for Environmental Infection Control in Health Care Facilities: Recommendations of CDC and the Healthcare Infection Control Practices Advisory Committee (HICPAC), *MMWR Morb Mortal Wkly Rep 52*(RR10), Jun. 6, 2003. http://www.cdc.gov/mmwr/preview/mmwrhtml/rr5210a1.htm (accessed Jun. 2, 2009).

Sidebar 6-2: Resources for Regulatory or Professional Guidelines

- American Institute of Architects, Academy of Architecture for Health, with assistance from U.S. Department of Health & Human Services: *Guidelines for Design and Construction of Hospital and Healthcare Facilities.* http://www.aia.org/aah_gd_hospcons.

- American Society of Heating, Refrigerating and Air-Conditioning Engineers: Handbook Series. *1999 Handbook—HVAC Applications,* I-P Edition: Chapter 7, Healthcare Facilities; Chapter 15, Clean Spaces; Chapter 44, Corrosion Control, Water Treatment. Also *1997 Handbook Fundamentals:* Chapter 9, Indoor Environmental Health; Chapter 12, Air Contaminants.

- Facility Guidelines Institute. http://www.fgiguidelines.org.

- National Fire Protection Agency: *Life Safety Code®* Handbook. National Fire Protection 101. http://www.nfpa.org.

- Water Quality Association. http://www.wqa.org.

- Association for Professionals in Infection Control and Epidemiology: Text of Infection Control and Epidemiology: Chapter 72, Construction; Chapter 73, Environmental Services; Chapter 74, Infectious Waste Management; Chapter 76, Maintenance and Engineering; Chapter 77, Ventilation; Chapter 78, Water Issues in Healthcare; Chapter 79, Occupational Health; Chapter 98, Legionella; Chapter 123 Disaster Response. http://www.apic.org.

- Sehulster L., Chinn R.Y.W.: Guidelines for Environmental Infection Control in Health Care Facilities. Recommendations of CDC and the Healthcare Infection Control Practices Advisory Committee (HICPAC). *MMWR Recomm Rep* 52(RR10), Jun. 6, 2003. http://www.cdc.gov/mmwr/preview/mmwrhtml/rr5210a1.htm.

The AIA guidelines do not describe or mandate how it is to be carried out, but merely require documentation that it was done to protect and prevent infectious risks to patients. One method, known as the ICRA Matrix, has been almost universally adopted because of its systematic approach to the process. Through 14 precise steps, it facilitates communication among clinicians, engineers, and architects. The ICRA Matrix is presented in Figure 6-1 on pages 88–93.

Construction and renovation are common in many facilities and pose some danger to immunocompromised and debilitated patients for various organisms. Events such as an absent or late IC risk assessment or a lack of appropriate barriers may warrant a high priority that identifies a particular area for improvement. Table 6-1 on page 93 provides generic examples by category for IC risk assessment.

Create a Multidisciplinary Process

What will be the outcome if the contractor fails to comply with specified IC practices? How will waste materials generated by the project be disposed of? Who decides if a patient/client/resident unit needs to close for the duration? These kinds of questions must all be decided before the health care organization gives a contractor the green light to begin a construction or renovation project.

A multidisciplinary team of professionals should be chosen by the organization, ensuring maximum input from all concerned parties and continuing coordination among affected departments. Typically ranging in size from just a few people for a minor renovation to close to 20 for construction of a new facility, the team should always include the person in charge of IC and may also include the following positions and disciplines:
- The facility manager
- Engineering
- Safety and risk managers
- The manager of employee health
- The architect
- Contractor representatives/construction managers
- Direct care supervisors
- Epidemiologist
- Environmental services
- Maintenance
- Housekeeping
- Environmental (airborne or waterborne) consultant

An organization's infection preventionist(s) should be involved in all phases of a construction project, starting with planning. For very high-risk projects, the organization might also consider hiring an outside expert in infectious material containment to work with the team.

Figure 6-1: Infection Control Risk Assessment Matrix of Precautions for Construction and Renovation*

Infection Control (IC) Risk Assessment
Matrix of Precautions for Construction & Renovation

Step 1:

Using the following table, identify the type of construction project activity (Type A–D).

TYPE A	**Inspection and non-invasive activities** Includes, but is not limited to: • Removal of ceiling tiles for visual inspection only, e.g, limited to 1 tile per 50 square feet • Painting (but not sanding) • Wall covering, electrical trim work, minor plumbing, and activities that do not generate dust or require cutting of walls or access to ceilings other than for visual inspection
TYPE B	**Small scale, short duration activities that create minimal dust** Includes, but is not limited to: • Installation of telephone and computer cabling • Access to chase spaces • Cutting of walls or ceiling where dust migration can be controlled
TYPE C	**Work that generates a moderate to high level of dust or requires demolition or removal of any fixed building components or assemblies** Includes, but is not limited to: • Sanding of walls for painting or wall covering • Removal of floor coverings, ceiling tiles, and casework • New wall construction • Minor duct work or electrical work above ceilings • Major cabling activities • Any activity that cannot be completed within a single work shift
TYPE D	**Major demolition and construction projects** Includes, but is not limited to: • Activities that require consecutive work shifts • Activities that requires heavy demolition or removal of a complete cabling system • New construction

Step 1

(continued on next page)

Figure 6-1: *continued*

Step 2:

Using the following table, *identify* the <u>Patient Risk</u> Groups that will be affected.

If more than one risk group will be affected, select the higher risk group.

Low Risk	Medium Risk	High Risk	Highest Risk
• Office areas	• Cardiology • Echocardiography • Endoscopy Nuclear • Medicine Physical Therapy • Radiology/MRI • Respiratory Therapy	• CCU • Emergency • Labor Room and Delivery • Laboratories (specimen) • Medical Units • Newborn Nursery • Outpatient Surgery • Pediatrics • Pharmacy Postanesthesia Care Unit • Surgical Units	• Any area caring for immunocompromised patients • Burn Unit Cardiac • Cath Lab • Central Sterile Supply • Intensive Care Units • Negative Pressure Isolation Rooms • Oncology • Operating Rooms including C-section Rooms

Step 2

Step 3:

<u>Match</u> the

Patient Risk Group *(Low, Medium, High, Highest)* with the planned

Construction Project Type *(A, B, C, D)* on the following matrix, to find the

Class of Precautions *(I, II, III or IV)* or level of infection control activities required.

Class I–IV Precautions are delineated on the following page.

IC Matrix—Class of Precautions: Construction Project by Patient Risk
Construction Project Type

Patient Risk Group	TYPE A	TYPE B	TYPE C	TYPE D
LOW Risk Group	I	II	II	III/IV
MEDIUM Risk Group	I	II	III	IV
HIGH Risk Group	I	II	III/IV	IV
HIGHEST Risk Group	II	III/IV	III/IV	IV

Note: Infection Prevention and Control approval will be required when the Construction Activity and Risk Level indicate that Class III or Class IV control procedures are necessary.

Step 3

(continued on next page)

Figure 6-1: *continued*

Description of Required Infection Control Precautions by Class

	During Construction Project	Upon Completion of Project
CLASS I	1. Execute work by methods to minimize raising dust from construction operations. 2. Immediately replace a ceiling tile displaced for visual inspection.	1. Clean work area upon completion of task
CLASS II	1. Provide active means to prevent airborne dust from dispersing into atmosphere. 2. Water mist work surfaces to control dust while cutting. 3. Seal unused doors with duct tape. 4. Block off and seal air vents. 5. Place dust mat at entrance and exit of work area. 6. Remove or isolate HVAC system in areas where work is being performed	1. Wipe work surfaces with cleaner/disinfectant. 2. Contain construction waste in tightly covered containers before transport. 3. Wet mop and/or vacuum with HEPA-filtered vacuum before leaving work area. 4. Upon completion, restore HVAC system where work was performed.
CLASS III	1. Remove or isolate HVAC system in area where work is being done to prevent contamination of duct system. 2. Complete all critical barriers—i.e., sheetrock, plywood, plastic—to seal area from nonwork area or implement control cube method (cart with plastic covering and sealed connection to work site with HEPA vacuum for vacuuming prior to exit) before construction begins. 3. Maintain negative air pressure within work site utilizing HEPA-equipped air filtration units. 4. Contain construction waste in tightly covered containers before transport. 5. Cover transport receptacles or carts. Tape covering unless solid lid.	1. Do not remove barriers from work area until completed project is inspected by the owner's Safety Department and Infection Prevention and Control Department and is thoroughly cleaned by the owner's Environmental Services Department. 2. Remove barrier materials carefully to minimize spreading of dirt and debris associated with construction. 3. Vacuum work area with HEPA filtered vacuums. 4. Wet mop area with cleaner/disinfectant. 5. Upon completion restore HVAC system where work was performed.
CLASS IV	1. Isolate HVAC system in area where work is being done to prevent contamination of duct system. 2. Complete all critical barriers—i.e., sheetrock, plywood, plastic—to seal area from nonwork area or implement control cube method (cart with plastic covering and sealed connection to work site with HEPA vacuum for vacuuming prior to exit) before construction begins. 3. Maintain negative air pressure within work site utilizing HEPA-equipped air filtration units. 4. Seal holes, pipes, conduits, and punctures appropriately. 5. Construct anteroom and require all personnel to pass through this room so they can be vacuumed using a HEPA vacuum cleaner before leaving work site, or they can wear cloth or paper coveralls that are removed each time they leave the work site. 6. All personnel entering work site are required to wear shoe covers. Shoe covers must be changed each time the worker exits the work area.	1. Do not remove barriers from work area until completed project is inspected by the owner's Safety Department and Infection Prevention and Control Department and is thoroughly cleaned by the owner's Environmental Services Department. 2. Remove barrier material carefully to minimize spreading of dirt and debris associated with construction. 3. Contain construction waste in tightly covered containers before transport. 4. Cover transport receptacles or carts. Tape covering unless solid lid. 5. Vacuum work area with HEPA-filtered vacuums. 6. Wet mop area with cleaner/disinfectant. 7. Upon completion restore HVAC system where work was performed.

(continued on next page)

Figure 6-1: *continued*

Step 4. Identify the areas surrounding the project area, assessing potential impact.

Unit Below	Unit Above	Lateral	Lateral	Behind	Front
Risk Group	Risk Group	Risk Group	Risk Group	Risk Group	Risk Group

Step 5. Identify specific site of activity, e.g., patient rooms, medication room, etc.

_____

Step 6. Identify issues related to ventilation, plumbing, electrical in terms of the occurrence of probable outages.

_____

Step 7. Identify containment measures, using prior assessment. What types of barriers (e.g., solids, wall barriers)? Will HEPA filtration be required?

_____

(Note: Renovation/construction area shall be isolated from the occupied areas
during construction and shall be negative with respect to surrounding areas.)

Step 8. Consider potential risk of water damage. Is there a risk due to compromising structural integrity (e.g., wall, ceiling, roof)?

Step 9. Work hours: Can or will the work be done during non–patient care hours?

Step 10. Do plans allow for adequate number of isolation/negative airflow rooms?

Step 11. Do the plans allow for the required number and type of hand-washing sinks?

Step 12. Do the infection prevention and control staff agree with the minimum number of sinks for this project?
(Verify against FGI Design and Construction Guidelines for types and area.)

Step 13. Does the infection prevention and control staff agree with the plans relative to clean and soiled utility rooms?

Step 14. Plan to discuss the following containment issues with the project team—e.g., traffic flow, housekeeping, debris removal (how and when).

_____

_____

_____

Appendix: Identify and communicate the responsibility for project monitoring that includes infection prevention and control concerns and risks. The ICRA may be modified throughout the project. Revisions must be communicated to the Project Manager.

(continued on next page)

Figure 6-1: *continued*

Infection Control Construction Permit					
				Permit No:	
Location of Construction:			Project Start Date:		
Project Coordinator:			Estimated Duration:		
Contractor Performing Work			Permit Expiration Date:		
Supervisor:			Telephone:		
YES	NO	CONSTRUCTION ACTIVITY	YES	NO	INFECTION CONTROL RISK GROUP
		TYPE A: Inspection, noninvasive activity			GROUP 1: Low Risk
		TYPE B: Small scale, short duration, moderate to high levels			GROUP 2: Medium Risk
		TYPE C: Activity generates moderate to high levels of dust, requires greater than 1 work shift for completion			GROUP 3: Medium/High Risk
		TYPE D: Major duration and construction activities requiring consecutive work shifts			GROUP 4: Highest Risk

CLASS I	1. Execute work by methods to minimize raising dust from construction operations. 2. Immediately replace any ceiling tile displaced for visual inspection.	3. Minor demolition for remodeling
CLASS II	1. Provide active means to prevent airborne dust from dispersing into atmosphere 2. Water mist work surfaces to control dust while cutting. 3. Seal unused doors with duct tape. 4. Block off and seal air vents. 5. Wipe surfaces with cleaner/disinfectant.	6. Contain construction waste in tightly covered containers before transport. 7. Wet mop and/or vacuum with HEPA-filtered vacuum before leaving work area. 8. Place dust mat at entrance and exit of work area. 9. Isolate HVAC system in areas where work is being performed; restore when work completed.
CLASS III **Date** **Initial**	1. Obtain infection control permit before construction begins. 2. Isolate HVAC system in area where work is being done to prevent contamination of the duct system. 3. Complete all critical barriers or implement control cube method before construction begins. 4. Maintain negative air pressure within work site utilizing HEPA-equipped air filtration units. 5. Do not remove barriers from work area until complete project is checked by Infection Prevention and Control and is thoroughly cleaned by Environmental Services.	6. Vacuum work with HEPA-filtered vacuums. 7. Wet mop with cleaner/disinfectant. 8. Remove barrier materials carefully to minimize spreading of dirt and debris associated with construction. 9. Contain construction waste in tightly covered containers before transport. 10. Cover transport receptacles or carts. Tape covering. 11. Upon completion, restore HVAC system where work was performed.
CLASS IV **Date** **Initial**	1. Obtain infection control permit before construction begins. 2. Isolate HVAC system in area where work is being done to prevent contamination of duct system. 3. Complete all critical barriers or implement control cube method before construction begins. 4. Maintain negative air pressure within work site utilizing HEPA-equipped air filtration units. 5. Seal holes, pipes, conduits, and punctures appropriately. 6. Construct anteroom and require all personnel to pass through this room so they can be vacuumed using a HEPA vacuum cleaner before leaving work site, or they can wear cloth or paper coveralls that are removed each time they leave the work site.	7. All personnel entering work site are required to wear shoe covers. 8. Do not remove barriers from work area until completed project is checked by Infection Prevention and Control and is thoroughly cleaned by Environmental Services. 9. Vacuum work area with HEPA-filtered vacuums. 10. Wet mop with cleaner/disinfectant. 11. Remove barrier materials carefully to minimize spreading of dirt and debris associated with construction. 12. Contain construction waste in tightly covered containers before transport. 13. Cover transport receptacles or carts. Tape covering. 14. Upon completion restore HVAC system where work was performed.

Additional Requirements:

Date	Initials	Date	Initials	Exceptions/Additions to this permit are noted by attached memoranda
Permit Request By:			Permit Authorized By:	
Date:			Date:	

(continued on next page)

Figure 6-1: *continued*

Steps 1–3. Adapted with permission from V. Kennedy, B. Barnard, St. Luke Episcopal Hospital, Houston, TX; C. Fine, CA.

Steps 4–14. Adapted with permission from Fairview University Medical Center, Minneapolis MN.

* MRI, magnetic resonance imaging; CCU, critical care unit; C-section, Cesarean section; HVAC, heating, ventilation, and air conditioning; HEPA, high-efficiency particulate air; FGI, Facility Guidelines Institute; ICRA, infection control risk assessment.

Source: Forms modified/updated and provided courtesy of Judene Bartley, Epidemiology Consulting Services, Inc., Beverly Hills, MI 2002. Updated 2009. Used with permission.

Table 6-1: **Generic Risk Categories and Risk Factors for Infection Prevention and Control (IC)**

Risk Categories	Risk Factors
Geographic Location	• Natural disasters: tornadoes, floods, hurricanes, earthquakes • Breakdown of municipal services: broken water main, strike by sanitation employees • Accidents in the community: Mass transit (airplane, train, bus) • Fires involving mass casualties • Intentional acts: bioterrorism, "dirty bomb," contamination of food and water supplies • Prevalence of disease linked with vectors, temperatures, other environmental factors
Community	• Community outbreaks of transmissible infectious diseases (influenza, meningitis) • Diseases linked to food and water contamination (for example, salmonella, hepatitis A) • Vaccine-preventable illness in unvaccinated population • Infections associated with primary immigrant populations in geographic areas • Public health structure • Socioeconomic levels
High-Risk Patients	• Surgical, intensive care unit, neonatal intensive care unit, oncology, dialysis, transplant, antibiotic resistance, multidrug-resistant organisms
Employee Risks	• Understanding disease transmission and prevention • Degree of compliance with infection prevention techniques and policies—hand hygiene, aseptic technique
Equipment and Devices	• Cleaning, disinfection, transport, and storage of equipment • Sterilization or disinfection processes
Environment Issues	• Construction, renovation, alterations • Utilities performance • Environmental cleanliness and safety
Emergency Preparedness	• Staff education • Managing influx of infectious patients • Utilities and supplies
Resource Limitations	• Infection prevention and control, staffing, environmental services

It should definitely bring charge nurses from the floors or units affected by the project into the process; in addition to providing critical insights into patient care needs, the more the team members know, the more helpful they can be in accommodating construction activities without compromising patient/client/resident care.

The risk assessment is only one of several elements for ensuring continuous input from IC into the structural design process. A construction and renovation policy could also include the routine submission of scheduled project lists from facility management to IC so that staff can better anticipate IC needs. It could also emphasize submission of an IC construction permit and the signatures of all parties, indicating accountability for the mutually agreed upon plan.

Health Care Worker Education

The organization and its leaders are responsible for providing or arranging for the education of project workers, both internal and external. Before construction starts, they need to know, at a minimum, about the following:

- How to adhere to IC measures and issues
- The potential risks associated with the project
- The use of particulate respirators or other personal protective equipment and how to use the equipment
- Risk prevention for safety issues, such as noxious fumes or asbestos
- How to seek help and report exposures

Workers should also receive pertinent health protection, which might include vaccinations and skin testing for tuberculosis. Contract agreements should provide evidence that worker education and protection measures have been taken.

Case Study 6-1 on pages 95-98 focuses on a five-year expansion project at The University Hospital in Cincinnati, where successful efforts to control and prevent infection depended on staff training and education. In addition, Case Study 6-2 on pagse 99-100 illustrates how construction design plays an important role in patient care room design.

Airflow

Airflow is always a top priority, as the most significant source of HAIs related to construction arises as a result of the dust raised during construction and demolition.[6] Preventing buildingwide contamination during construction requires careful planning because all buildings have some degree of recirculation in their ventilation systems. Air must flow from clean to dirty areas. The HVAC engineer must determine how to isolate the system, which might include tactics such as sealing vents and adding additional filters.

An airborne infection isolation room (AIIR), also referred to as a negative pressure isolation room, is a single-occupancy patient care room used to isolate persons with a suspected or confirmed airborne infectious disease. Environmental factors are controlled in AIIRs to minimize the transmission of infectious agents that are usually transmitted from person to person by droplet nuclei associated with coughing or aerosolization of contaminated fluids. AIIRs should provide negative pressure in the room (so that air flows under the door gap into the room); an air flow rate of 6 to 12 air changes per hour (ACH; 6 ACH for existing structures, 12 ACH for new construction or renovation); and direct exhaust of air from the room to the outside of the building or recirculation of air through a HEPA filter before returning to circulation.[7]

Table 6-2, page 101, outlines engineered specifications for positive- and negative-pressure rooms.

Negative air machines, capable of drawing in and filtering up to 2,000 cubic feet of air/minute or more, function like a fan using a built-in filter and exhaust system. HEPA–filtered units can filter out 99.97% of particulate matter. Make sure that the point of discharge is not in a public pathway; this might mean removing a window panel and installing a temporary panel with a duct opening in it.

In small-scale projects, such as running wires above a ceiling, workers can build a plastic cube around the work area and put it under negative pressure with a small negative air unit or a HEPA–filtered vacuum cleaner, exhausting the air outside the cube. Note that conventional shop vacuums are not up to this job, allowing both dust and fumes back into the air. An IC checklist that can be used by EC professionals is illustrated in Figure 6-2, page 101.

Case Study 6-1: Quality Improvement: Establishing Collegiality and Trust Among Health Care Staff and Contractors

Organization Facts

The University Hospital (TUH) is a large tertiary-care hospital in Cincinnati, Ohio. As part of the Health Alliance of Greater Cincinnati, it has a level 1 trauma center, seven intensive care units (including a level 3 perinatal research center and neonatal intensive care unit), an adult burn unit, and comprehensive outpatient services with 450,000 visits per year. TUH admits more than 26,000 patients per year and has 85,000 emergency room visits.

Project Description

TUH expanded and codified its infection prevention and control (IC) training program for contractors due to a major renovation project. The IC staff, in-house design and construction staff, and outside contractors met before the initiation of all major renovation projects to predict any IC-related concerns and to proactively plan for interventions. A team was established to monitor and recommend continuous improvements during the renovation project. All contractors and maintenance staff were required to receive IC training at the time of employment, a stick was affixed to the hospital identification badge to indicate the IC training date, and staff members were educated about IC-related construction concerns so that staff could help monitor airflow and cleanliness.

Outcomes

TUH's contractors remained compliant with IC specifications, construction and maintenance staff contacted the IC program to obtain advice, and there were 4 years of extensive construction without any hospital-acquired *Aspergillus* infections due to changes to the IC program.

Effective infection prevention and control (IC) depend on trust, cooperation, education, and collegiality among staff. Because the health care–associated infection (HAI) caused by *Aspergillosis* is disseminated by hospital construction and renovation,[1] IC compliance must be expected not only of hospital staff, but it must also be expected from contractors and construction workers during short- and long-term renovations, demolition, construction, and maintenance. Although IC requirements for construction projects had been previously established at The University Hospital (TUH) in Cincinnati, ground-level construction-site workers tended not to comply with IC requirements due to a lack of information and understanding. In response to a major hospital renovation, TUH proactively expanded and codified an extant IC training program for contractors.

Background

In 1994, an outbreak of *Aspergillosis* infections in heart transplant units at TUH prompted construction restriction policies, and the IC program added *Aspergillosis* surveillance to its targeted program. In January of 2000, TUH began a new five-year construction project to expand an existing operating room (OR) and add a nine-story garage, postanesthesia care unit, and cardiothoracic intensive care unit. TUH sought to reduce risk to immunosuppressed patients by increasing IC compliance through an expanded IC education program.

Ensuring Patient-Safe Demolition and Construction

Before construction could begin, five buildings, circa 1910, had to be demolished.[2] Since *Aspergillus* spores are stirred up and can enter patient care areas,[1] safe demolition was the first necessary phase of the new construction project. The following precautions were taken:

- Windows in patient rooms were sealed with plastic.
- Staff monitored prevailing wind and added additional prefilters to all air intakes.
- Dust generated by demolition was wetted down.
- Air curtains were added to doorways facing construction.
- Immunosuppressed patients were instructed to wear N95 protection when entering the facility.

(continued on next page)

Case Study 6-1: *continued*

When old buildings were demolished, particulate samples were taken in high-risk areas in order to measure the effects of new interventions.

When construction began, each construction site was contained in an effort to keep all construction dust from infiltrating patient care areas. Essentially, each construction site was surrounded with barriers and negative airflow was maintained. The air pressure inside the construction area was lower than the air pressure outside of the construction area. This way, dust generated by the job and within the barriers could not leak out into patient care areas (*see* Sidebar 1, below).

Expanding the IC Education Program

To effectively comply with IC and protect immunosuppressed patients, all construction site staff needed to understand the reasons behind IC construction requirements. Hence, continuing to emphasize the interdisciplinary nature of education for hospital staff and contractors was a fundamental component of expanding the IC construction model program.

Prior to 2000, the IC education program had established the need for education about construction and IC. When the 2000 construction project began, the current TUH hospital manager was knowledgeable about interventions needed to protect immunosuppressed patients, as well as management of indoor air quality during construction projects. In addition, members of the hospital's design and construction department were engineers and architects who had attended classes on construction and IC. However, although general contractors were aware of IC construction requirements, there was no in-depth understanding of the need for compliance. Frontline workers had even less information.[2]

Assembling Multidisciplinary Teams

IC teams were established that included a general contractor, project manager, IC professional, and/or nurse planner. These teams visited project sites on a weekly basis and helped coordinate difficult scenarios as they arose. For example, when contractors had to walk through the heart transplant OR to get to the project site, the team established procedures to make sure patients were protected (*see* Sidebar 2, page 97).

(continued on next page)

Sidebar 1. Precautions for Construction Site Adjacent to Patient Care Areas

The multidisciplinary infection prevention and control (IC) team established the following procedures to protect immunosuppressed heart transplant patients:

- Anterooms were built for contractors to change between clean and dirty sites.

- Workers were required to wear hair covers, shoe covers, and bunny suits over their clothing as they passed through the operating room (OR).

- Airflow gauges monitored negative airflow, and OR staff were taught to read airflow gauges.

- OR staff were taught how to respond if airflow was positive.

- Contractors wet-mopped floors throughout the workday to avoid tracking of construction dust.

- Workers did projects off-hours whenever possible.

- An IC professional inspected and approved barriers before construction commenced.

- An IC professional had the authority to stop a project in case of a breach in practice/precautions.

- An IC professional developed an open-door policy to address any questions or concerns from construction site workers, plumbers, maintenance staff, and so on.

- A disciplinary process was developed for noncompliant construction site workers.

- Renovation and construction contracts included verbiage outlining IC behavior and practices expected from all contractors and construction site workers.

- Written explanation of IC construction site constraints and a corresponding written test were developed for one-time or short-term construction site workers.

- An IC professional regularly visits construction sites with a particulate-meter to measure efficiency of interventions and barriers around construction sites.

Case Study 6-1: *continued*

Education Method

The new IC training program requires that all TUH construction and maintenance personnel receive yearly IC education training conducted by the project manager and attended by an IC employee. The 30-minute education class explains how *Aspergillus* is transmitted and that immunosuppressed patients are particularly vulnerable. The class includes precautions that must be taken before, during, and after construction work is executed. The emphasis is on containment of construction dust including ceiling access, high-efficiency particulate air filtration, barriers, establishing negative airflow, and using tacky walk-off mats. For short-term (for example, one-day or one-visit) construction/maintenance work, staff are required to read education materials and take a written test.

All construction staff wear mandatory hospital identification badges indicating that the education training has been completed. Workers who have not completed the training can be identified by sight, and the badge precludes discussion about lack of information or excuses if a construction worker is not following precautions.

IC professionals visit all projects weekly; large projects are visited daily by IC teams. During weekly meetings, team members discussed potential adjustments to interventions and precautions. During site visits, the IC team and IC professionals had authority to stop any project if there was a breach in IC policy or precautions.

Overcoming Obstacles

Initial resistance to change was founded on the perception that complying with IC precautions took too much time. A three-step disciplinary process was developed to address noncompliance. The first instance of noncompliance results in a verbal warning, the second results in a written warning, and the third results in either a fine or dismissal. Architects and engineers in the design and construction department are assigned as construction managers. Periodic and occasionally unannounced visits from IC staff also help ensure compliance.

Despite some initial resistance, classes and regular site visits helped develop a sense of trust and congeniality over the course of a project. Discussions and an open-door policy by IC staff help maintain effective communication among hospital staff and construction site workers. In addition, the formal justification and reasons for IC policies eliminate any personal issues from conflicts or noncompliant behavior that may arise.

(continued on next page)

Sidebar 2. The University Hospital Infection Control/Construction Model Program

Guidelines for an infection control/construction model program might include the following:

- Develop and document a carefully considered policy.

- Involve infection prevention and control (IC) personnel from the initial stages of the construction project.

- Use IC risk assessment before beginning the construction project.

- Identify any and all IC conditions in the construction specifications.

- Educate and train all workers including all construction managers and supervisors.

- Provide all workers with identification badges indicating IC training designation.

- Issue permits for special tasks that could contribute to patient risk.

- Ensure team quality assurance by IC, project managers, contractors, and hospital staff.

- Monitor airflow and confirm that the project area is negative to patient care.

- Consider particulate sampling to establish a record of dust contribution.

- Investigate construction sites adjacent to the hospital to determine outside sources of particulates.

- Maintain IC involvement by providing approval of barriers and inspections.

- Establish that the project manager and IC are authorized to stop the project.

- Involve all hospital maintenance staff.

- Cultivate collegiality among all involved.

Case Study 6-1: *continued*

Results

Results of TUH's IC construction program were statistically significant. In the first four years of the five-year project, no patients acquired nosocomial *Aspergillus* infections. Two patients with a possible HAI were identified during the fifth year of construction. Particulate sampling was repeated and levels had not changed since the old buildings had been demolished. IC staff found that both patients acquired infections when a connected nonhospital building began a renovation project without using IC techniques.

As a final step in the process, two key players, an IC professional and staff engineer working on the OR project, wrote up the program and experience under the tutelage of the hospital epidemiologist in order to share their successes and struggles with other hospitals facing similar challenges.

Ongoing IC of Construction Sites

IC staff held meetings with administrators of the adjacent building that leaked *Aspergillus* into patient care areas. TUH contractors helped educate contractors of the adjacent building; all contractors worked together to establish negative airflow within the adjacent building.

Since the new IC training program was implemented, IC professionals continue to streamline and develop the education curriculum. An IC professional meets with the design and construction department for monthly meetings to address additional improvement opportunities. For example, the hospital has now formalized the process of removing "dead legs"—stray pieces of pipe in the water supply system—that can collect water and foster the growth of microbials. In addition, the IC professionals responsible for visiting construction sites regularly measure the particulate level of the air around the perimeter of sites to ensure that particulate levels are at or below average.

References

1. Cooper E., et al.: Influence of building construction work on *Aspergillus* infection in a hospital setting. *Infect Control Hosp Epidemiol* 24(7):472–476, 2003.

2. Kidd F., et al.: Construction: A model program for infection control compliance. *Am J Infect Control* 35(5):347–350, 2007.

Case Study 6-2: Modern Hospital Design for Infection Prevention and Control

In the past, hospital design focused on low cost per square foot or the incorporation of new technology, and was based on models of nursing care derived from industrial settings where the transmission of infection was not a consideration. For example, placing two or more patients close to each other would seem to be more efficient for nursing care, as this would require that nurses take fewer steps between patients and would minimize square-footage requirements. In this model, the patient was considered to be like a product requiring assembly by the staff.

Organization Facts

Bronson Methodist Hospital (BMH) is a large nonprofit tertiary-care hospital in Kalamazoo, Michigan, serving all of southwest Michigan and northern Indiana. BMH has 380-beds in private rooms and provided inpatient services to 23,509 patients in 2008. BMH provides care in virtually every adult and pediatric specialty and is a regional destination for trauma and critical care. BMH has been recognized for many quality achievements including the 2005 Malcolm Baldrige National Quality Award.

Project Description

In 2000, BMH replaced its older, primarily semiprivate-room hospital with a new facility incorporating private rooms. In the semiprivate room design, two patients shared the room and a bathroom, and most hospital rooms did not have a dedicated hand-washing sink for staff; staff members used the patient bathroom to wash their hands. The private room design makes the spread of infection

Outcomes

In the new private room design, each patient room has a bathroom and a separate hand-washing sink in a convenient location for staff use. During the first four years of the project, no patients acquired Aspergillus infections.

Newer design models incorporate the patient's perspective and are based on medical-outcome evidence, patient satisfaction, and patient safety. One of the most important shifts in hospital design in the past few years has been to design patient-care spaces for infection prevention and control (IC).

Treatment of patient infections comprises a significant percentage of the operational costs of any hospital. Many patients are admitted with infections or with diseases that make them more susceptible to infection, and without proper IC, infections can spread among patients and staff. Standard hospital cleaning procedures[1] and standards for air and water systems[2] have reduced the risk of infection from the hospital environment; hence, very few health care–associated infections come from the building's air or water. Today, the primary source of hospital-spread infections is personnel who move from patient to patient, often carrying medical devices and equipment. Modern hospitals should be designed to reduce this risk of transfer of infection by personnel.

Semiprivate room designs increase the likelihood of infections spreading among patients and staff. Private rooms make the spread of infection less likely because patients and visitors do not share space and equipment with other patients.

An important factor in the transmission of infection is proximity, and one of the most effective ways to reduce the risk of transmission is to increase the functional distance between patients. Open ward or semiprivate room designs make it more likely that infections can be spread among patients and staff.

Patients carry microorganisms on their bodies, and patients with infections can shed increased numbers of infection-causing microorganisms. The items surrounding the patient (bed, furniture, equipment, and so on) become

(continued on next page)

Case Study 6-2: *continued*

contaminated with the patient's microorganisms after he or she spends more than a few hours in his or her room. The most common way infections are spread is by staff members touching a patient or contaminated piece of equipment with their hands, then touching another patient without washing their hands. Hand hygiene is the single most important way to prevent hospital infections, and the current Centers for Disease Control and Prevention hand-hygiene guidelines[3] clearly mandate that all health care personnel decontaminate their hands as they enter a patient's room and as they leave the room. Locating a dedicated hand-washing sink, preferably with hands-free operation, near the door of each patient room makes staff hand hygiene easier and contributes to a safer environment for patients, staff, and visitors.

Methodology

Bronson hypothesized that the rate of infection would be reduced in its new facility and designed a study to test that hypothesis. Bronson measured the rate of health care–associated infections monthly in its old, semiprivate units for two years before the opening of its new hospital and compared those rates with the two-year period following occupation of its new, private-room hospital. Bronson did not change its nursing staff or patient-care model, the number of beds and patient volume did not change significantly, and the types of patients and their diagnoses did not change significantly during this period.

Findings

The total health care–associated infection rate among all patient care units in the new facility declined 11% (from 0.89 to 0.80 infections per 1,000 patient days), as measured monthly for 24 months in the old facility and for the first 24 months in the new facility. Among the six patient care units that changed from a semiprivate to a private room design, the infection rate declined by 45%, a statistically significant difference. The infection rates in the critical care units that did not change from a semiprivate to a private room design also declined, but the difference did not reach statistical significance. This reduction translated to five fewer infections or four fewer infected patients per month in the new facility. This study showed that the infection rate was reduced in the private-room facility and suggested that the reduction was because of the private-room design.

The study did not measure staff hand-hygiene compliance during the comparison period, so we could not determine if the reduction in infection was because of reduced proximity or increased hand hygiene by staff. It is likely that both factors contributed to the safer environment.

Discussion and Conclusions

Because infections significantly add to the cost of medical care, reductions in infection rates significantly reduce the operational costs of the hospital and the overall costs of medical care, as well as make the hospital a safer environment for the patient. The reduction in operational costs due to a lower infection rate alone should pay for the additional construction costs of the private-room design and produce a positive return on investment in only a few years.

References

1. Schulster L., Chinn R.Y.W.: Guidelines for Environmental Infection Control in Health-care Facilities: Recommendations of CDC and the Healthcare Infection Control Practices Advisory Committee (HICPAC). *MMWR Morb Mortal Wkly Rep* 52(No. RR-10), 2003.

2. American Society of Heating, Refrigerating and Air-Conditioning Engineers (ASHRAE): Report of the Presidential Ad Hoc Committee for Building Health and Safety Under Extraordinary Incidents. Washington, D.C.: ASHRAE, 2003.

3. Centers for Disease Control and Prevention: Guideline for Hand Hygiene in Health-care Settings: Recommendations of the Healthcare Infection Control Practices Advisory Committee and the HICPAC/ SHEA/APIC/IDSA Hand Hygiene Task Force. *MMWR Morb Mortal Wkly Rep* 51(No. RR-16), 2002.

Special thanks to Richard A. Van Enk, Ph.D., C.I.C., Director of Infection Control and Epidemiology at Bronson Methodist Hospital, Kalamazoo, MI, for his invaluable assistance with and contributions to this case study.

Table 6-2: Engineered Specifications for Positive- and Negative-Pressure Rooms

Specification	Positive Pressure Area	Negative Pressure Area
Pressure differentials	> 2.5 Pascal (0.01" water gauge)	> p2.5 Pascal (0.01" water gauge)
Air changes per hour	> 21	> 12 (for renovation or new construction)
Filtration efficiency	Supply: 99.97% @ 0.3 μm dioctylphthalate particles; exhaust: none	Supply: 90% (dust spot tests); exhaust: 99.97% @ 0.3 μm dioctylphthalate particles
Room airflow direction	Out to the adjacent area	Into the room
Clean-to-dirty airflow in room	Away from the patient (high-risk or immunosuppressed patient)	Toward the patient (airborne disease patient)
Ideal pressure differential	> 8 Pascal	> 2.5 Pascal

Note that these specifications are recommendations rather than requirements. Individual organizations will want to consult with engineering staff or consultants to develop their own specifications.

Source: Centers for Disease Control and Prevention: *Guideline for Environmental Infection Control in Health Care Facilities.* 2003. http://www.cdc.gov/ncidod/dhqp/gl_environinfection.html (accessed Jan. 11, 2009).

Figure 6-2: Infection Prevention and Control Checklist for Construction/Renovation

Project: _____

Reviewer: _____ Date: _____ Time: _____

	Yes	No	N/A	Comments
Are temporary construction barriers dust tight?				
Are temporary hole penetrations in walls and ceilings covered adequately?				
Are ceiling tiles replaced at end of shift if removed for access?				
Are doors kept closed or appropriately sealed?				
Has existing ductwork been covered or sealed?				

Source: Soule B., Kitchin D.: Working together: Infection control & EOC/life safety. Presented at The Joint Commission Resources/Continuous Service Readiness Program, Little Rock, AR, Jun. 2008.

Facility-Specific Final Tasks

Constructing a checklist of facility-specific final tasks to work through before beginning construction is important. The following generic checklist might be suitable:

☐ Set the path of entry and exit from the construction zone to the staging area outside of the facility.

☐ Place appropriate signage to keep patients/clients/ residents, health care staff, family, and other visitors away from area and path.

☐ If an elevator must be used to access the construction zone, key off one elevator car from public or staff use to access the work zone.

☐ Set up an anteroom around the designated elevator to prevent dust and debris from contaminating the elevator shaft.

☐ Provide tacky mats at the entrance to construction anteroom and construction zone.

☐ Identify the HVAC system for the construction zone and develop a way to isolate the system from the zone, such as cutting out both the supply and return air grills.

During Construction

Precautions to take during construction involve checking on safety measures put in place before construction. For example, after setting up tacky mats and designated exit and entry paths, an organization will want to monitor the site to make sure workers are using and changing them regularly. In the same way, monitors should check that all materials leaving the construction zone and the facility itself are securely bagged and placed in covered rollout bins and that materials coming in are handled the same way.

Workers often wear disposable coveralls, sometimes known as bunny suits, in the construction zone. These coveralls should stay in the zone. Workers can leave them in the anteroom before accessing the cafeteria, restrooms, or any other nonconstruction areas in the facility—assuming that the contract specifically grants such access.

Although no regulatory agencies currently recommend that organizations routinely take environmental cultures during construction, the ICRA should outline targeted patient/ client/resident surveillance near construction areas, for example, for respiratory illnesses consistent with the highly lethal airborne fungus *Aspergillus*.

Aspergillus species are found in decaying cellulose, water, and dust, and spread based on the following:

• Spores that attach to dust particles and then spread in the air

• Tolerates almost any temperature

• Needs two to three days to grow in water

Fungi, such as *Aspergillus* species, tend to grow in the main spaces of construction and in finishing materials, such as porous materials in damp locations.

Another contaminant that construction activity is likely to stir up is the bacteria *Legionella*. This gram-negative, aerobic, rod-shaped bacterium is found in natural aquatic environments, as well as in soil and dust.[8] During construction and renovation projects, water systems are often disrupted, and the potable water can become contaminated with *Legionella* when the water supply is restored. *Legionella* can proliferate in the facility's water supply if certain conditions exist, such as sediment in hot water tanks, low hot-water temperatures at faucets, and water systems that are prone to stagnation.

The occurrence of an infection caused by *Legionella* depends on the resistance of the individual, exposure to a contaminated source, and the degree of contamination of the source. Therefore, preventive measures to decrease the transmission of *Legionella* should be implemented when construction or renovation activities that disrupt some of the health care facility's water supply are planned.[8]

In addition, construction or renovation can be counted on to generate a lot of inorganic nuisance and respirable dust that can cause eye and throat irritation, among other discomforts, and fibers that affect mucous membranes.

After Construction

IC measures taken at the completion of a construction project are just as important as those applied in preparation of a project. In fact, the time to establish postconstruction agreements is well before construction gets underway to ensure that all debris and construction dust from ceiling cavities, wall cavities, vertical shafts, and utility chases involved in construction are properly removed and all surfaces in the construction zone—including ceilings, walls, cabinets, partitions, and flooring—are properly cleaned.

Cleanup Agreements

Among the agreements the health care organization should have in place are cleanup agreements covering, at a minimum, the following responsibilities[9]:

- Contract cleaning that includes clearing the area, cleaning, and decontamination and wiping down surfaces
- Cleaning after removal of partitions around construction area
- Facility-based routine cleaning before the area can be occupied by others
- Creating time frames for review after completion of the project
- Systematic review of outcomes ranging from sealed cabling and electrical penetrations and ceiling tile replacements to a completed punch list
- Cleaning and replacement of filters and other equipment if affected by major or minor conditions that could have contaminated the air or water supply

The walk-through just before occupancy should follow a similar project-specific checklist that answers key IC questions, including such questions as the following:

- Are sinks properly located and functioning?
- Do sinks in critical care areas have properly functioning fixtures?
- Are soap and towel dispensers filled and working?
- Are surfaces in procedure and service areas appropriate for use?
- Has air balancing been completed according to specifications?
- Does air flow into negative pressure rooms and out of positive pressure rooms?

References

1. Smith C.E.: GREENGUARD: Why challenges of indoor air in hospitals are different. *Sustainable Facility*, Aug. 2007. http://www.sustainablefacility. com/CDA/Articles/Greenguard/BNP_GUID_9-5-2006_A_10000000000000146359 (accessed Jun. 11, 2009).

2. Bartley J.: Hospital construction: stirring up trouble. *Engineered Systems Magazine*, Jul. 1, 2007. http:// www.esmagazine.com/Articles/Feature_Article/BNP_ GUID_9-5-2006_A_10000000000000126814 (accessed Jun. 11, 2009).

3. American Institute of Architects: *Guidelines for Design and Construction of Health Care Facilities*. http://www.aia. org/aah_gd_hospcons (accessed Jun. 11, 2009).

4. Schulster L., Chinn R.Y.W.: Guidelines for Environmental Infection Control in Health Care Facilities: Recommendations of CDC and the Healthcare Infection Control Practices Advisory Committee, Centers for Disease Control and Prevention (CDC). *MMWR Morb Mortal Wkly Rep* 52(RR10), Jun. 6, 2003. http:// www.cdc.gov/mmwr/preview/mmwrhtml/rr5210a1.htm (accessed Jun. 11, 2009).

5. Agency for Healthcare Research and Quality: *Transforming Hospitals: Designing for Safety and Quality*. http://www.ahrq.gov/qual/transform.htm (accessed Jun. 11, 2009).

6. From Construction to Infection. *Hosp Manage*, Sept. 10, 2007. http://www.hospitalmanagement.net/features/ feature1351/ (accessed Jun. 11, 2009).

7. Jensen P.A., et al.: Guidelines for Preventing the Transmission of *Mycobacterium tuberculosis* in Health Care Settings. *MMWR Recomm Rep* 54(RR17), December 30, 2005. http://www.cdc.gov/mmwr/ preview/mmwrhtml/rr5417a1.htm (accessed Jun. 11, 2009).

8. Health Canada: *Construction-Related Nosocomial Infections in Patients in Health Care Facilities: Decreasing the Risk of Aspergillus, Legionella and Other Infections*. Canada Communicable Diseases Report, vol. 2752, Jul. 2002. http://www.phac-aspc.gc.ca/publicat/ccdr-rmtc/01pdf/27s2e.pdf (accessed Jun. 11, 2009).

9. Noskin G.A., Peterson L.R.: Engineering infection control through facility design. *Emerging Infectious Diseases* 7, Mar.–Apr. 2001. http://www.cdc.gov/ncidod/ eid/vol7no2/noskin.htm (accessed Jun. 11, 2009).

Emergency Management

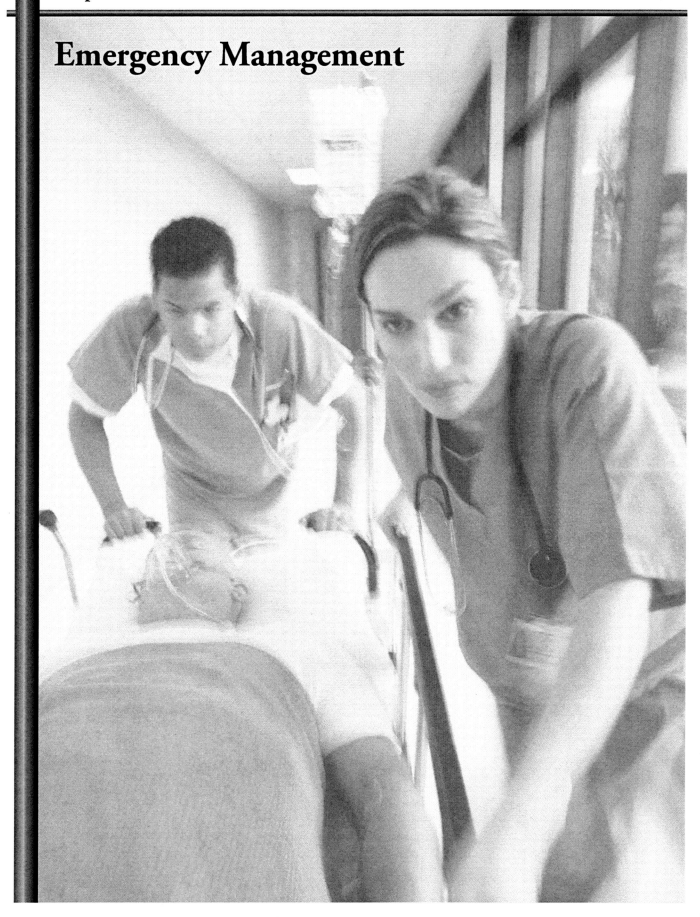

Emergency Management

Since the September 11, 2001 terrorist attacks, U.S. hospitals and other types of health care organizations have become increasingly active in planning and coordinating a facility- and community-based response to major emergencies—whether natural, such as Hurricane Katrina and Hurricane Ike, or human-made, such as a bioterrorist attack. Recognizing this, The Joint Commission added infection prevention and control (IC) and emergency management (EM) standards explicitly requiring facilities to prepare to respond to an influx of infectious patients. This chapter outlines the procedures and requirements of an IC and environment of care (EC) EM plan, and explores integral EM aspects, such as preparedness for surge capacity, the role of the facility manager in the EM plan, conducting decontamination planning, and recommended measures in the decontamination of facilities.

The Emergency Management Plan

The EM plan is leadership-driven, but all health care staff members are involved. Now more than ever, IC and EC professionals must work together to prepare for any influx of patients.

In the event of a major emergency that brings a sudden surge of patients to a health care facility, EC and IC leaders and staff play a particularly important role in planning for the provision of critical supplies and equipment, security, isolation and decontamination facilities, communications systems, building utility systems (for example, electricity, water, ventilation, fuel sources, medical gas/vacuum systems), and alternative care sites. A problem with any one of these elements can significantly impact an organization's ability to handle even normal—not to mention catastrophic—surges in patient flow.

Indeed, the most fundamental component of the organization's EM plan might be *surge capacity*—the organization's ability to expand care capabilities in response to sudden or more prolonged demand.

Determining Surge Capacity

Surge capacity has both a point-in-time aspect (that is, the ability to accommodate patients for a limited time period during the acute crisis) and a longitudinal dimension (the ability to manage longer term care needs.) It encompasses the following elements[1]:

- Potential patient beds
- Available space in which patients can be triaged, managed, treated, vaccinated, decontaminated, or simply located
- Available personnel of all types
- Necessary medications, supplies, and equipment
- Legal capacity to deliver health care services under situations that exceed authorized capacity

According to the Centers for Disease Control and Prevention (CDC), in 2006 the nation's emergency physicians treated more than 119.2 million visitors to the emergency department (ED).[2] On any given day, many hospitals are struggling to meet the current demand for services. Handling mass casualties or a pandemic on top of the daily patient load would be difficult, at best.

And what if the mass casualties are infectious? The rationale for the IC standard stresses that the organization is an important resource for the continued functioning of a community. As such, it must plan how to prevent the introduction of the infection into the organization, how to quickly recognize that this type of infection has been introduced, and how to contain the spread of the infection if it is introduced.

Acting on concerns about the juncture of surge capacity and IC, the Florida Agency for Health Care Administration investigated ways to expand the surge capacity of Florida hospitals to cope with infectious disease outbreaks. Hospitals were alerted to deal with the following scenarios:

- How to manipulate the hospital's heating, ventilation, and air conditioning (HVAC) system to turn patient rooms into negative air rooms and exhaust this negative infectious air to the outside without returning it to the building

- How to find products that can be affixed to walls or ceilings to convert normal patient rooms into negative air rooms
- How to set up a temporary structure within a designated area of the community that would enable a certain segment of the population to be isolated

A working group at Tampa General Hospital submitted the following guidelines to the Florida Hospital Association for review by and input from other hospitals throughout the state with the eventual hope to enact these recommendations to regulate patient placement and movement in case of a disease outbreak:

- The facility will accommodate 10 beds.
- The facility has negative air pressure in relation to surrounding areas.
- The facility will provide a magnahelic gauge to ensure that pressure differentials are maintained.
- The facility is monitored continuously for negative air pressure.
- The facility will provide at least 12 air changes per hour of circulation (supply and exhaust).
- Air is exhausted to the outdoors on the roof of the facility through monitored high-efficiency particulate air (HEPA) filters; no air from this facility is circulated to other areas.
- Supply air is conditioned for summer or winter.
- The facility will provide automatic door closers to ensure that doors are closed.
- The facility will provide anterooms with air supply to maintain positive air pressure.
- The facility will provide medical gas (oxygen, vacuum, and medical air) at each bed.
- The facility will provide an emergency power supply to critical medical equipment and air circulation equipment.
- The facility will provide hand hygiene facility and toilet facility.

Hazard Vulnerability Analysis

Hospitals following the Joint Commission EM standards complete a hazard vulnerability analysis (HVA) to identify in advance potential emergencies that could affect the need for their services or their ability to provide those services. This analysis provides an opportunity to set up pre-established supplier relationships for the identified vulnerabilities.

Recommendations for the Facility Manager

The following is a list of recommendations for hospital facilities managers culled from suggestions by Susan Kwolek, vice president of quality and corporate performance at

North York General Hospital, Canada, and by Lucy Brun, a Toronto-area health care and infectious disease expert:

- Provide sufficient surge capacity to address emergencies.
- Reduce the number of entry and exit points to the facility; control access via cameras and swipe cards.
- Separate the hospital's "mission-critical" departments and access to these areas.
- Increase the number of isolation rooms that include technique anterooms and three-piece washrooms.
- Implement mechanical and ventilation systems to support isolation and separation of air intakes and exhaust.
- Provide adequate individual space per patient; for example, more than four feet from one patient or visitor face to the next patient or visitor face.
- Keep an adequate supply of personal protective equipment (PPE; face masks, gloves, gowns, and so on) on hand at all times and make sure that those supplies are readily available.
- Clean patient units on every shift.
- Clean all facilities and equipment that are in common use, such as nursing stations, computer keyboards, telephones, and so on.
- Use basic IC methods as outlined in the Joint Commission standards in the applicable accreditation manual.
- Consult the Web site of the CDC at http://www.cdc. gov/page.do, which has a section devoted to severe acute respiratory syndrome (SARS) at http://www.cdc.gov/ ncidod/sars/ and at http://www.cdc.gov/ncidod/sars/ guidance/I/index.htm.

Sidebar 7-1, page 109, lists other threats for facility managers and other staff to be aware of. Sidebar 7-2, page 109, lists questions to ask concerning influenza outbreak and anthrax exposure.

Conducting Decontamination Planning

In the event of an IC emergency, the Joint Commission standards require that acute care hospitals, critical access hospitals, ambulatory care, and long term care organizations make arrangements to decontaminate persons affected by toxic radioactive, biological, and chemical substances. Note that all these organizations need not actually have decontamination facilities themselves, but it is currently considered advisable for acute care and critical access hospitals.

Decontamination Efforts

For their part, ambulatory care and long term care organizations will want to work within the community to determine where decontamination activities will occur.

Sidebar 7-1: Other Threats and Questions to Consider

Public health officials consider severe acute respiratory syndrome to be the first severe and readily transmittable disease of this century. But many other diseases have been identified in recent decades. Organizations will want to consider these in their emergency management plans. Among them are the following:

- Bioterrorism agents (chemicals and biologics such as smallpox)
- Dengue fever
- Food-related outbreaks (such as *E. coli*)
- Malaria
- Methicillin-resistant *Staphylococcus aureus*
- Norwalk
- Vancomycin-resistant enterococci
- Chicken pox
- Ebola
- Influenza
- Meningitis
- Multidrug-resistant tuberculosis
- Other respiratory viruses (such as respiratory syncytial virus, parainfluenza)
- West Nile virus
- Anthrax

Sidebar 7-2: Questions to Ask About Influenza and Anthrax

Influenza Outbreak

- How will your organization handle a larger crisis in the community if all its emergency department (ED) beds are filled with victims of influenza?
- Why are ED beds filled with victims of influenza? What education might be provided communitywide to reduce use of the ED in the event of a flu outbreak?
- How might immunization in the community be enhanced?
- What contingency plan does your organization have if adequate quantities of flu vaccine are unavailable?

Anthrax Exposure

- What criterion does your organization use to determine whether and when to implement emergency management procedures for a known or possible bioterrorist exposure?
- What criteria does your organization use to determine when to contact appropriate local, county, state, and federal agencies of a possible bioterrorist contamination? Is contact information for each of these agencies kept in a central location and known to all?
- How is your organization's bioterrorist response integrated with local fire, police, and public health departments?
- What physical measures would your organization take to prepare the facility and your staff for a large influx of possibly contaminated victims?
- What provisions would your organization make in the event that staff cannot enter the facility due to contamination?
- Have you made provisions for areas of your facility that could be converted to additional care areas for possibly contaminated victims? How will airflow and water systems be contained?
- How and to where would decontamination capabilities expand in the event of a mass contamination? How will you ensure reasonable privacy for victims?
- What criteria will your organization use for deciding whether decontamination procedures are indicated and what tests, if any, need to be performed?
- What provisions have been made to secure and protect the facility from contaminated victims entering without being decontaminated?
- Have provisions been made for the loss of services, functions, or areas as a result of contamination?
- What provisions are in place for containing, securing, and returning victims' clothing and valuables?
- How would the social service needs of victims (clothing, pharmaceuticals, food, and so forth) be met?

Such activities would involve isolating the contamination; decontaminating and treating victims; protecting staff, other patients, visitors, and the facility itself; and effectively reestablishing normal service. In preparing for this type of emergency, organizations should identify where contaminated victims will be housed, as well as how and where they will be decontaminated and how the organization will handle and store the variety of contaminated materials.

It should be noted that decontamination is primarily used in cases of chemical or radioactive contamination. The first recognition of an unannounced biological incident might occur when symptomatic victims present themselves in the ED, following an unknown incubation period. At that point, decontamination would serve no purpose. It would be useful, however, for victims who arrive at the facility actually covered with the substance in question.

Sometimes a hospital gets a warning of a hazardous materials release or exposure. If notified in advance that it will be seeing victims of such an incident, hospital officials should communicate this information up the chain of command and confirm it with the local emergency management services (EMS) authority. The initial call taker at the hospital should record the following essential pieces of information:

- Type and nature of the incident
- Callback number to obtain updates
- Name of the chemicals involved
- Symptoms being experienced
- Any associated conditions (burns, trauma)
- Total number of patients anticipated
- Degree of contamination, if any, performed at the scene

The number of patients needing decontamination will vary with the nature of the incident. Some information and forewarning can come through contacts with the EMS agencies, but the full hazard potential of the incident might not be known for several hours. Most of the potential victims will be triaged to area hospitals in the first two to three hours, and many will arrive without the help of the local EMS system. However, isolated cases with delayed symptoms that come into local EDs might be difficult to connect with a hazardous materials release. Sidebar 7-3, right, offers signs of symptoms.

Sidebar 7-3: Symptom Signs

Certain clinical signs and symptoms should lead emergency department staff to suspect that persons have been exposed to hazardous materials, most noticeably nausea, dizziness, itching or burning of the eyes or skin, and cyanosis. If any of these show up repeatedly, it is important to alert the community command post, which can in turn alert personnel at the scene to look for signs of hazardous materials release. Unanticipated contaminated patients can quickly move through and contaminate a hospital during an emergency, possibly requiring the hospital to close until it is decontaminated.

TIP: Develop a plan to respond to an influx of patients over an extended period of time.

Strategy: Although handling an influx is important, organizations also need to be prepared for an epidemic that takes place over an extended period. For example, the 2003 SARS outbreak lasted from February 10, 2003, to July 5, 2003, when the World Health Organization deemed it to be contained. By that time, the number of confirmed cases worldwide had reached approximately 8,500, with more than 900 dead. Organizations should consider the following issues when developing a response plan:

- Staffing: Will the organization be able to maintain sufficient staff over a period of months to care for patients? How will the hospital cope with the very real possibility of staff who become exhausted by the demands of patient care?

- Quarantine: Will the organization's staff members need to be quarantined? If so, will they be quarantined at home? At work? How will the organization help staff members cope with extended absences from their families and/or coworkers?

- Supplies: How will the organization acquire the equipment and supplies it needs to continue functioning, such as food, medications, clean water, and air filters?

- Finance: How will the organization be reimbursed for caring for large numbers of infectious patients?

If there are multiple patients arriving for decontamination, the principles of triage apply. The priorities for providing medical care for contaminated victims should follow this order:

1. Life-threatening conditions
2. Primary assessment together with contamination reduction
3. Thorough decontamination
4. Secondary survey
5. Hazardous materials identification

Occupational Safety and Health Administration Requirements

As required by the Occupational Safety and Health Administration (OSHA), decontamination procedures should be performed at the first triage station, and decontamination equipment should be easily accessible. Invasive procedures, unless required by a life-threatening condition, should be deferred until decontamination is finished because they can serve as portals of entry for the contaminating material.

It is important to remember that as soon as victims are decontaminated, they can be treated as normal patients and triaged to the most appropriate patient treatment area for definitive care. The medical staff should be aware that some substances can produce significant delayed effects, so a sound strategy will include prolonged observation, frequent reevaluations, and patient monitoring.

Equipment Decontamination

In addition to decontaminating people, organizations should have a plan for decontaminating equipment. Some equipment is easy to clean. Other items, such as permanent negative air equipment, will present more challenges. The plan should reference arrangements with a state-approved hazardous waste contractor for removing contaminated materials produced during the decontamination process.

Note that although some hospitals have long assumed that the fire department will be responsible for decontamination, it might be involved at the scene of the event and thus not available for this function. Furthermore, in small incidents such as agricultural or garage accidents, individuals might present themselves in the ED without warning, and the hospital will need to perform appropriate decontamination procedures without waiting for outside assistance.

In addition to meeting the Joint Commission standards on IC, hazardous materials, safety, and participation in

TIP: Meet with all departments—both clinical and nonclinical—to plan how your organization will handle its resources if it needs to accept an influx of infectious patients.

Strategy: Determine whether you want to continue providing services in case of an epidemic, and if so, how you can do this. The following are some questions to consider for handling ongoing patient care:

- Will the purchasing department need to identify auxiliary suppliers for infection control and prevention, such as masks, gowns, and gloves?

- Where will you get the equipment you'll need in order to provide negative air pressure in patient rooms?

- Will you need to provide housing and meals for staff members who are quarantined at their jobs? Would you be capable of furnishing child-care services for their family members?

- Will you need to expand your housekeeping staff to meet the enhanced cleaning standards required during an outbreak?

- What kind of training and rehearsals will be needed to prepare staff for coping with an influx of infected patients?

TIP: EC professionals and infection preventionist should work together to plan how your organization will respond in the event of an influx of infectious patients.

Strategy: Determine which functions will need to be performed in response to an outbreak and which individuals or departments will be responsible for those functions. Create a list of essential departments that will need to be accessible and/or operational during an influx of infectious patients.

Strategy: Map out a brief but relevant written plan to identify critical needs. List the strategies to meet those needs. Crafting a response plan is essential to minimize harm to patients and staff members alike.

Strategy: In addition, review your facilities management plans to identify critical infrastructure that must function during an outbreak. Proper sanitation measures are vital in containing the spread of infection, not just among the general public, but also among health care workers who treat infectious patients. To prevent the spread of infection, the Centers for Disease Control and Prevention (CDC) issued specific technical recommendations on cleaning and disinfection of environmental surfaces, environmental sampling, laundry and bedding, and regulated medical waste in its Guidelines for Disinfection and Sterilization in Healthcare Facilities, 2008.[1]

communitywide planning, a victim decontamination program has numerous other benefits—such as protection of staff, minimization or elimination of facility contamination, and protection of key areas from abandonment. Another benefit is the financial savings that result from avoiding the financial burdens of cleanup costs, revenue-affecting shutdowns, and fines from regulatory agencies. The ability to decontaminate and treat chemically contaminated persons is a benefit to the community as well as the workplace, in that employees who become contaminated might otherwise have to be transported to another facility, putting their own colleagues in danger while waiting for transport.

Decontamination Facilities

Decontamination facilities may be internal to the facility as long as they have a direct entrance from the outside and a separate ventilation system that exhausts directly to the exterior of the building. Alternatively, a number of portable decontamination units for outside use can also be effective, even in colder climates. There are pros and cons to both.

When considering where to locate the decontamination area, it is important to note that with many chemical incidents, the primary problem is the chemical vapors. Approximately 80% of the contamination is removed with the victim's clothing. Design plans must spell out where victims will disrobe, what they will cover themselves with after decontamination, and how their original clothing will be packaged, all of which will help avoid further exposures of patients and staff.

TIP: Determine who in your organization will be responsible for staying abreast of current information on IC.

Strategy: If your organization does not have staff that focus exclusively in IC, such as an infection preventionist or an epidemiologist, assign a staff member or develop a committee to monitor information about disease outbreaks and prevention measures, as well as recent developments in preventing and treating infectious diseases. In coping with outbreaks of infectious diseases, your organization can access a wealth of communication channels to help you stay up-to-date and informed. Among the many sources for information are 24-hour radio news stations, broadcast television, and cable channels. Many organizations have Web sites where they post the latest information about outbreaks and IC tactics. In addition, check with your local health department as well as the CDC for up-to-date information on IC.

Given the significant likelihood that a portion of the facility itself will be contaminated and need to be quarantined, organizations should evaluate their layouts to determine whether the air handling systems can be isolated to prevent the spread of contaminants throughout the building, and whether certain rooms, corridors, or entrances might be used to isolate or quarantine staff and patients.

Equipment such as fire-rated plastic sheeting, duct tape, and spring-loaded poles can be used to cordon off hallways or other areas and separate contaminated areas from clean ones, although this plan might be difficult to do in a small facility. Again, small facilities might determine that they are not appropriately equipped to handle such emergencies and choose to work instead within the community to combine resources.

In setting up a decontamination area, there should be a dirty side and a clean side. The dirty side, where all victims and contaminated personnel and equipment should stay until decontaminated, should include a triage station, treatment station, and decontamination area, the latter able to accommodate both ambulatory and nonambulatory victims. Victims should perform as much of the decontamination as possible to decrease cross-contamination.

If air respirators are selected as PPE for the health care workers, the room or outdoor area should be designed with multiple connections to a dedicated air compressor or a bank of compressed air tanks. Alternatively, as long as patient care is not compromised, the respirators can be connected to the piped medical air system.

The decontamination area should be large enough to accommodate at least one stretcher patient and the requisite decontamination team members, including the following:

TIP: Determine how you want to distribute whatever information you receive from public health sources.

Strategy: Make a list of the appropriate departments within your organization that will receive relevant information about disease outbreaks, including the primary and secondary information recipients. For example, how soon should the clinical departments be notified so they can call in extra staff? At what point should the organization notify nonclinical departments such as facilities management, housekeeping, and security about an action alert?

- An emergency physician
- ED nurses and aides (the number depending on the number of victims)
- Support personnel, including a nursing supervisor, an occupational health and safety officer, a security staff member, a maintenance staff member, and someone to provide documentation

Sidebar 7-4, right, provides information on decontamination team training.

There has been extensive debate in the health care community about the appropriate level of PPE for decontamination activities. Current consensus is that Level C provides adequate protection. This level means chemical resistant and splash proof, with chemical-resistant gloves and boots and either a full- or half-face air-purifying respirator. Respirators are available with stacked cartridges to address organic vapors and acid gas and to provide HEPA filtration, which is effective against most chemical agents that terrorists might use.

Outdoor Decontamination Facilities

Outdoor facilities have the advantage of keeping the contaminant totally outside the health care facility. Portable units for outdoor use are available that cost less than brick and mortar construction, even if multiple units are required. On the other hand, it takes time to set up the units, and it is imperative that this part of the process be drilled to reduce the time as much as possible.

Other types of outdoor facilities utilize plumbing on the outside of the building. There might be a sheltered area near the ED, perhaps in a corner or other type of protected space where showerheads can be installed on the exterior and connected to the facility's normal water supply. This system retains the advantage of an outdoor facility and eliminates the time factor required to set up a portable unit.

Climate is a definite consideration in contemplating an outdoor decontamination facility. However, even in colder climates, an outdoor facility can be strategically located in an area adjacent to the building and connected to hot and cold running water sources. A functional system can be designed with the exit of the unit in close proximity to the entrance of the building and with a staff member waiting there with blankets for the victim.

Outdoor facilities do pose a privacy problem, which must be given serious consideration. There has been successful

---

Sidebar 7-4: Decontamination Training

In selecting staff to perform decontamination, health care organizations should consider recruiting those who might already have a basic knowledge of hazardous materials and emergency response—security, housekeeping, plant operations, and other staff who are volunteer firefighters, emergency medical technicians, or paramedics. Clinical staff should also be involved in the decontamination program because they will be able to medically assess victims during the process.

The organization's policy and procedures should address decontamination training in line with the mandate by the Occupational Safety and Health Administration to provide operations training for those who will be involved in the actual decontamination. At a minimum, all emergency department employees should have an understanding of victim decontamination issues.

Organizations should train staff to recognize possible hazardous situations and to respond properly and immediately. It is important to focus the training on identifying victims who might have come in contact with biological or chemical agents and on avoiding contamination of the facility and staff to avoid having to impose a shutdown or quarantine.

Organizations that can assist with training include the Environmental Protection Agency (EPA), which provides a four-hour care recipient decontamination program that can be offered without cost (http://www.epa.gov).

Although the organization's first priority is to ensure victim, patient, and staff safety, team members can also be trained in procedures that aid in epidemiological investigation, ongoing surveillance, or criminal investigation.

TIP: Assign responsibility to specific people in your organization for contacting local and regional health departments.

Strategy: Many local public health organizations are set up to send health care alerts, share information, and foster collaboration among the public health, medical, and emergency communities in their area. Ask local health departments to add your organization's name and contact information to the list of those who will receive fax or e-mail alerts about disease outbreaks.

legal action by victims who underwent a decontamination process without regard for their privacy. Many victims needing decontamination might not otherwise be injured and therefore can essentially decontaminate themselves with a soap and water shower. They need to have a private place to disrobe and deposit their contaminated clothing, and males and females must be separated.

The EPA requires that, under manageable circumstances, water used for decontamination be collected and analyzed for hazardous materials prior to disposal. In very large events, the EPA has acknowledged that care of victims is of primary importance, with containment of the water a secondary issue. Portable decontamination units typically have bases that contain the water; however, if they are used for multiple victims, there might be overflow. Another way to contain the water is to have the victim stand in an inexpensive children's swimming pool. Systems plumbed directly from the building could also use a drain to a holding tank.

Indoor Decontamination Facilities

Indoor decontamination facilities obviously overcome any climate concerns and have easy access to plumbing, but their location poses other problems, among them the need to avoid contamination of the ED or the facility as a whole. In addition, they cannot as easily accommodate multiple victims. Then, too, with space at a premium in hospitals, an empty room is a vacuum waiting to be filled, and indoor facilities must be ready for use at all times.

Required supplies and equipment should be easily accessible, but cabinets and other similar storage spaces should be avoided because the room itself will need to be easily decontaminated following use. A sealed container, such as a metal drum, should be available for disposal of contaminated items.

There should be absolutely no traffic of contaminated individuals through the building. This is a difficult concept in itself, in that a victim might appear at the registration desk with no warning. If notified in advance, however, organizations can use outdoor triage that allows individuals to enter directly into the decontamination facility.

An indoor facility should be maintained at negative pressure from the ED, which might require additional equipment. Exhaust should be directed outside to avoid contaminating other parts of the facility.

Water collection is also an issue in indoor facilities. A tank placed below a drain in the floor to catch the used water should hold around 500 gallons to accommodate several victims and enable workers to draw samples for testing. Depending on the results, the water might either be discharged to the sewer or pumped out (or otherwise collected) for appropriate disposal. Again, children's pools can be used.

It is important to ensure that water is contained within the room itself, typically with the use of a floor pitched away from the door and toward the drain. Some facilities use dikes at the doors, which do the job but make it impossible to move victims via gurney. Once victims are decontaminated in an indoor facility, they should proceed through another doorway into the treatment area in the ED.

TIP: Develop a plan for communicating critical information to all staff.

Strategy: Communication is a key element in responding to an influx of patients, infectious or otherwise. The emphasis here is communicating with all staff in the organization. Create a plan showing when and how to reach the people who will need to provide clinical and nonclinical services. Maintain a list of staff members' phone numbers, both landlines and cell phones, as well as other communication devices. As part of your plan, prepare to answer the following questions nonclinical staff members might ask:

- How long might we be needed?

- What arrangements should we make to be away from home?

- What health risks will we face while on duty?

TIP: Identify your information resources, both internal and external.

Strategy: Consult with other organizations that have already created their own plans in order to determine what kind of events to plan for and what to address in your own response plan. Consider the following:

- How much information will you release to the media about changes in your patient population?

- How will you release that information? Through in-person interviews on radio and/or television? Press briefings? Press releases? How often will you release that information?

- How will you respond to inquiries from the patients' family members about the status of their loved ones? Who will be the information liaison?

References

1. Joint Commission Resources (JCR): Health Care at the Crossroads: Strategies for Creating and Sustaining Communitywide Emergency Preparedness Systems. Oakbrook Terrace, IL: JCR, 2003, p. 19.

2. Centers for Disease Control and Prevention: National Hospital Ambulatory Medical Survey: 2006 Emergency Department Summary. National Health Statistics Reports 7, Aug. 2006. http://www.cdc.gov/nchs/data/nhsr/nhsr.008.pdf (accessed Jun. 5, 2009).

Performance Measurement and Improvement

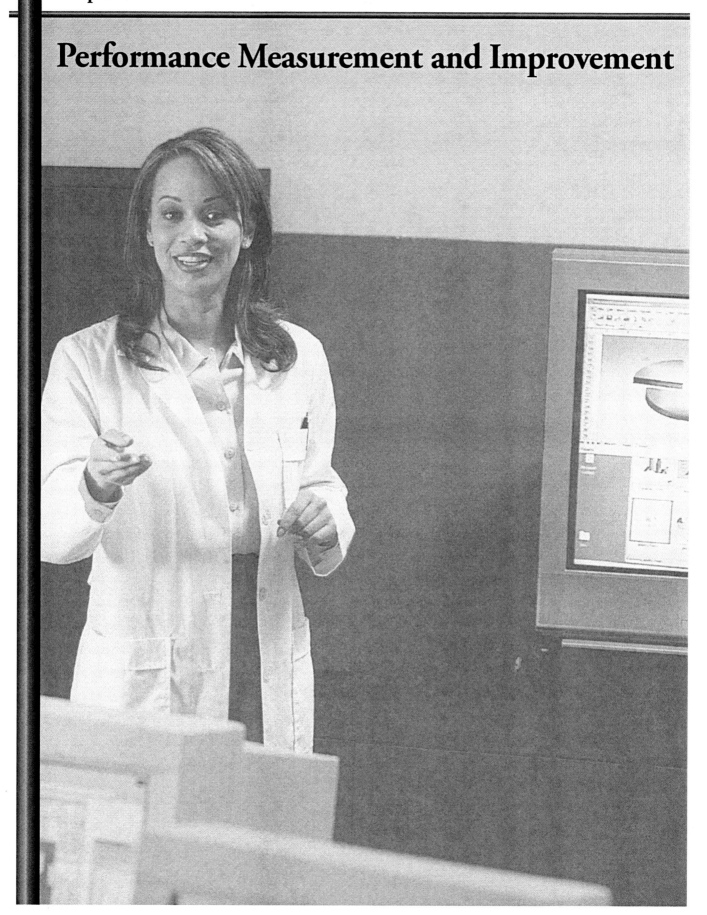

Performance Measurement and Improvement

Performance improvement (PI) is central to Joint Commission accreditation. Priority focus areas (PFAs)—defined as processes, systems, and structures that significantly impact the safety and quality of care—are the framework for the accreditation process. Thus, the 14 PFAs that The Joint Commission has identified to date make a good starting place for PI initiatives. One of the 14 is infection prevention and control (IC).

Measurement helps assess level of performance, determine whether improvement actions are necessary, and ascertain whether improvement has occurred. It allows organizations to assess the strengths and weaknesses of its systems and processes. Measure a process properly and you can use the information to improve patient safety, health outcomes, patient perceptions of care quality, and resource use associated with care.

A Teamwork Approach

Teams are particularly popular vehicles for PI. Although naturally occurring work teams such as employees within a single department are sometimes used to study a problem or complete a project, leaders more often assemble interdisciplinary teams and, particularly in the PI context, charge them with the responsibility of understanding and improving the performance of one or more dimensions of an important function, process, or outcome. To achieve a balanced perspective on the team, all functional areas related to the purpose and scope of the improvement project should be represented (*see* Case Study 8-1, pages 121-124).

The Joint Commission standards require organizations to analyze identified environment of care (EC) issues and take action on the identified opportunities to improve the EC. This includes establishing and following a multidisciplinary process, having a multidisciplinary improvement team meet at least bimonthly to address EC issues, and establishing measurement guidelines. The standards also call for appropriate staff to evaluate changes to determine if they resulted in improvements, and require that the organization report PI results to those responsible for analyzing EC issues.

As we have seen in earlier chapters, IC issues intersect with several of the key EC management plan areas—in

particular safety, hazardous (infectious) materials, emergency management, medical equipment, and utilities. Therefore, PI efforts in these areas will often involve collaboration between IC and EC leaders. PI would be enhanced with inclusion of leaders from clinical and support services.

In addition to actually developing and implementing or arranging for implementation of improvement strategies, such PI teams may also have a role in the following tasks:
- The ongoing collection of information about deficiencies and opportunities for improvement in the environment
- The ongoing collection and dissemination of other sources of information, such as published hazard notices or recall reports
- The preparation of summaries of deficiencies, problems, failures, and errors related to IC in the EC
- The preparation of summaries on findings, recommendations, actions taken, and results of PI activities

The way in which an interdisciplinary team works together has much to do with the success or failure of its efforts. Before the team can function effectively, it must master basic concepts of communication and collaboration. Nowhere is this more important than on IC/EC improvement teams, in which people often have different levels of interpersonal skills and varied knowledge and expertise about their specialty areas, and might be from different cultures. Team leaders should ensure that the following communication pieces are firmly in place on all such teams:
- All participants understand the project's overall objectives.
- Participants understand their roles and responsibilities as well as their relationship to other staff members.
- Participants take the time to establish and clarify guidelines and procedures for a working relationship.
- Participants define and agree on meaningful and measurable objectives that meet both group and personal needs.
- Participants function well in a variety of roles—initiating, informing, summarizing, mediating, encouraging—and know when each is needed.

What to Measure

The standards require that organizations establish and implement a process for ongoing monitoring of performance regarding actual or potential risks in each of the EC management plans. An example of risk might include failure to maintain the proper number of air exchanges in protected environment (PE) rooms and specialty areas such as operating rooms (ORs), setup of portable decontamination facilities that exceeds desired time limits, or too frequent spills involving infectious materials.

In addition to during annual reviews of EC management plans, risks might be identified as part of a failure mode and effects analysis (FMEA) of a given process, during the root cause analysis (RCA) of a sentinel event or near miss (*see* Case Study 8-2, pages 125-127) in a suggestion submitted by a staff member or a complaint registered by a patient or family member, as a result of new information in the literature, or in the course of routine monitoring. And, of course, investigations triggered by outbreaks or clusters of health care–associated infection (HAI) are also likely to identify appropriate targets for PI initiatives.

Fortunately, most health care organizations experience very few outbreaks or even individual incidents specifically related to the EC. This does not mean that performance measurement and improvement must wait on such an event (*see* Case Study 8-2). Instead, traditional forms of surveillance used to track and evaluate data relating to actual infections must be augmented by regular collection and analysis of data on process measures. These are measures that ask, "Are we doing what we said we were going to do? Are we adhering to our own policies and procedures?"

The following are some examples of process measures that organizations might monitor to stay on top of elements in the IC program that are grounded in the EC:

- What percentages of maintenance and housekeeping employees have been vaccinated for hepatitis B?
- Do employees involved in reprocessing reusable instruments wear appropriate personal protective equipment (PPE)?
- Are temperatures in refrigerators used for medicines and foods recorded according to schedule?
- Are negative pressure isolation rooms actually under negative pressure?
- Are linen carts covered as appropriate?
- Have all contract workers been trained in general and specific IC concepts and strategies?

- Are housekeepers changing their cleaning cloths as often as called for in policy?
- Are emergency eyewash stations flushed weekly?
- Are items to be sterilized prepared and packaged properly?
- Are items of PPE such as gloves available in a full range of sizes and types?
- Are ice machines being cleaned according to manufacturers' instructions?

If the answer is no, what corrective actions can be taken to bring the situation in line with expectations? If the answer is yes, is this the best the organization can do, or should expectations be raised? Just as important is the follow-up question: How do we know this answer is correct? That is, how is the organization validating and documenting the information? For example, if staff are educating visitors in isolation rooms about hand hygiene and proper use of PPE, are these interactions being documented? Do reprocessing logs reflect the number of times sterilizing equipment is tested?

Collecting Data

In many cases, collecting performance data is a matter of simple observation, often aided by the use of checklists. Two particular forms of observation are popular with many organizations, as follows:

- Environmental rounds, also called walking rounds, are similar to periodic environmental tours but may be performed more often by the EC and IC staff. These rounds provide an opportunity to collect concurrent and prospective data on an ongoing basis. For infection preventionists, these may occur during regular surveillance activities and provide the opportunity to discuss both clinical and environmental issues with the staff. The rounds may also include review of charts, laboratory reports, antibiotic use, and culture reports that will identify HAIs that may be related to environmental issues. EC personnel also make these rounds and collect data on selected environmental processes or facility infrastructure and can combine them with their regularly scheduled quality monitoring of equipment and utilities. Both the infection preventionist and the EC staff can use this opportunity to interview other staff to determine their understanding of disease transmission and their role in preventing infection. Point (or "period") prevalence is a way of taking a snapshot of the entire organization in a single day or other defined brief time period—visiting every room to check on a whole range of measures, such as high dusting, appropriate signage and storage, and so on.

Case Study 8-1: Process Improvement: The Mock-Up Room and Infection Prevention and Control

In building a 308-bed facility at the University Medical Center at Princeton (UMCP), leadership, caregivers, patients, and non-clinical staff including cooks and housekeeping are collaborating to design the safest possible facility and patient rooms. As of Spring 2009, and after years of planning, construction of the new facility has begun. All elements of design are based on evidence-based practices to prevent injuries and infection including consideration of human factors engineering to increase compliance with infection prevention and control (IC) policies. The environment of care—including the design, selection, and placement of rooms and their furnishings and medical equipment—can make significant contributions to IC, particularly in protecting patients from health care–associated infections (HAIs).[1]

Organization Facts
University Medical Center at Princeton (UMCP), a unit of Princeton HealthCare System, is a 308-bed acute care hospital located in New Jersey. UMCP integrates its care with advanced technologies, diagnostics, and treatment protocols. UMCP is also a member of the Association of American Medical College's prestigious Council of Teaching Hospitals and Health Systems. The new facility will consist of 636,000 square feet of interior space on 50 acres, with designated centers of care for cancer, surgery, testing and treatment, neuroscience, emergency, maternal child health, eating disorders, and cardiac and pulmonary care.

Project Description
The new hospital is being built using the latest in green building techniques. The mock-up room is designed to monitor risks of infection at every step of the care process so that an effective IC plan can be implemented in the new facility.

Outcomes
The mock-up room will allow UMCP staff to discover unanticipated effects of different designs and technology on infection prevention and control.

Before the new Princeton facility is complete, an integral part of the process will involve experimentation with a mock-up room on one of the current facility's nursing units. Designing and experimenting with a mock-up room is a multi-phased process (*see* Sidebar 1, page 122) emphasizing ongoing risk assessment and monitoring at every step of the process—a strategy essential to an efficient and effective IC plan.

Phases of the Mock-up Room
Experimenting with the design of a mock-up room and emphasizing patient safety and IC involves, at a minimum, four intensive phases. Although preliminary planning for the facility was led by a steering committee including the CEO, senior management, consultants, and caregivers, design and experimentation of the mock-up room was driven by caregivers as opposed to administrators and leadership. However, by the final phase of the mock-up process, experimentation and information gathering will have involved the following:
- Consultants
- Contractors
- Patients and their families
- Caregivers, including nurses, physicians, and respiratory therapists
- All non-clinical staff including dieticians, housekeeping staff, and building maintenance

Involving a multidisciplinary body such as the above will draw expertise from many sources, and raise awareness and commitment to preventing infections organizationwide.

In the first phase of designing the mock-up room, a foam-board version has been set up off site for pre-design research. This is the phase in which UMCP staff are currently involved. Caregivers are experimenting with bed rails, sink and hand-sanitizer placement, distance from the bed to the bathroom, light switches, sharps containers, storage for personal protective equipment, and other medical equipment. For example, caregivers will be testing to make sure sinks do not disappear behind bathroom or patient room doors and remain directly in the caregiver's work path.1 In addition, caregivers will be designing the foam- board room for maximum efficiency; a perceived

(continued on next page)

Case Study 8-1: *continued*

lack of time or the need to leave the room for equipment and supplies can increase the chance that a nurse fails to perform hand hygiene after contaminating her hands from the room and equipment to the patient, or vice versa.

After reviewing design possibilities and having discussions about the experiences of phase one, the room is built with plywood and caregivers simulate procedures. During phase two, caregivers will admit fictitious patients and ensure that the physical design of the room encourages compliance with IC. For example, the following will be considered:

- Are glove dispensers at an appropriate height and location to facilitate use?
- Does the room need two sharps containers rather than one?
- Is there sufficient clearance from opening and closing doors and supply cabinets to maintain an open work path with access to personal protection equipment and hand sanitizers?

In phase three, the actual room will be built on the nursing unit, and additional simulation will be performed. For example, the room might be intentionally infected with bacteria in a particular location. After a fictional patient is admitted, staff will investigate the room for spread of the bacteria and examine how it may have been spread (for

example, through direct or indirect contact, water source, and so on). In addition to investigating the cleanability and durability of surfaces and building materials, staff will investigate whether the sink splashes water. Studies have found that sink drains—a source of contaminants and HAIs such as Pseudomonas aeruginosa—can infect patients and contaminate the room if the sink does not contain spray/splashing from the faucet.[2]

During phase four, real patients are admitted into the model room. Staff will collect data and gather information about the patient and family experience, incidence of falls, and so on. In terms of IC, if an infected patient is admitted to the facility, caregivers will be able to check the room after the patient has been discharged in order to understand how or whether the infection has contaminated the room and equipment. In this way, meaningful performance measures will be included before the new facility is completed and its patient rooms are constructed.

Human Factors and IC

Although design features of the mock-up room will contribute to a culture of safety, several design features integrate IC directly. Perhaps foremost is that the mock-up room—and rooms in the new facility—will be a private patient room. Private patient rooms isolate infected patients or patients who may acquire an infection during their stay. Evidence-based that UMCP staff have based this decision on indicate that double and multi-bed rooms are significantly inadequate for preventing spread of some infections. In addition, private rooms are easier to decontaminate.[1] Because evidence-based research shows that the highest rates of infection occur in ICU patients[1], private ICU rooms will be designed with two sinks—one in the caregiver zone and an additional sink further into the room.

In terms of hand hygiene, working in a private room eliminates the temptation to move quickly from one patient bed to another without washing hands, and research indicates that private rooms may promote handwashing.[1] Overall, there is the possibility that fewer persons will enter the patient room if it is a private room rather than double or multiple patients room. In addition, staff has decided to use a nurse server in each room. Using a decentralized,

---

Sidebar 1. Phases of the Mock-Up Room

Designing and building a mock-up room for minimizing risk of infection in patient rooms is a multi-step process that includes the following:

Phase One: Caregivers experiment with a foam board version of the room set up off-site

Phase Two: Caregivers experiment with a plywood mock-up room and simulate procedures with fictional patients

Phase Three: The actual mock-up room is built in the current facility that involves experimentation and testing of equipment, building materials, and simulated procedures with fictional patients.

Phase Four: Real patients use the room. Information is gathered about the patient experience, caregiver experience, incidence of falls, infection rates, and so on

(continued on next page)

Case Study 8-1: *continued*

locked storage cabinet including 99% of the medical equipment and supplies needed for each room will help IC in several ways, including the following:

- Minimizes the number of staff/persons entering and exiting the patient room, possibly without performing hand hygiene
- Ensures that policies and procedures for sterilizing and storing medical equipment are followed
- Reduces or eliminates the need for nurses to leave the room looking for supplies, which may decrease hand hygiene by a perceived lack of time, and may also increase the chance of the nurse carrying germs in and out of the patient room

In addition to point of care supplies in a nurse server, the mock-up room will include personal protection equipment in an appropriate location (not hidden behind doors or outside of the work path), hands-free sinks and sanitizer dispensers, and technological reminders to perform hand hygiene. Such technology may involve flashing lights, beeping, or voice reminders. The multidisciplinary team will experiment with several options (*see* Sidebar 2, right).

In part, the experience of designing a mock-up room in phases will allow the team to make discoveries about unanticipated effects of different designs and technology. Therefore, it will be important for all team members involved to communicate and collaborate across the spectrum of care during simulations and when real patients and their families are using the room. It will be as valuable to hear from patients and their families about the comfort of the room as from housekeeping staff regarding what is easiest to clean and what equipment or horizontal surfaces may be hidden behind opened doors during routine cleaning.

Designing for Flexibility

In terms of efficient and effective IC, facility and patient-room design must be flexible and built with possible outbreaks and surges in mind. Particularly, the IC policies and practices must be maintained during such times. According to plans for the new facility, and in keeping with Princeton HealthCare System's IC, emergency department rooms will also be private, and unlike the current facility where space is constrained, there will be no hallway beds. Although the state of New Jersey does not require having all

Sidebar 2. Minimizing the Risk of Infections

Design features of a patient room that can minimize the risk of infection and infection transmission include the following:

- Private patient rooms
- Hands-free faucets, hand sanitizer dispensers, paper towel dispensers, and so on
- Splash-free sink
- Personal protection equipment (such as gloves) at an appropriate height and location
- Technological reminders—such as flashing lights or beeping—to remind caregivers to perform hand hygiene upon entering a patient room
- Installation of nurse servers/point of care cabinets to minimize the number of persons entering the patient room
- Selecting building materials (such as drawers and surfaces) with rounded corners to prevent cracks that can accumulate dirt and germs
- Cleanability of surfaces, such as non-cloth furniture or seamless sealed floors

respiratory isolation rooms on a unit in case of an outbreak, staff are discussing the possibility, as well as the possibility and need for building more isolation rooms than the Department of Health requires.

Looking Ahead

When the mock-up room is built in its final phase, IC professions will be able to vigorously measure infection rates before and after the new design. Throughout and beyond all phases, including the move-in to the new facility in 2011, staff will continue to evaluate and test best practices, both as part of its own learning and design process as well as in order to make meaningful contributions to a growing body of evidence-based research.

(continued on next page)

Case Study 8-1: *continued*

Designing the Patient Room: An Evidence-Based Approach to Creating a Healing Environment for Patients and Staff

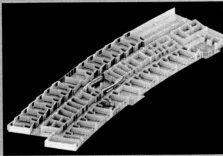

■ Patient unit axonometric

Components necessary to create a healing environment:
■ psychologically supportive environments
■ patients sense of control
■ social support
■ positive distractions
■ reduced negative distractions

Mock up Room
The University Medical Center at Princeton will be building a functional mock up room in the existing hospital which will be used for 2 years prior to the opening of the replacement hospital. Functional mock up rooms provide an opportunity for caregivers, patients, visitors and all members of the healthcare team to actually utilize the proposed room design prior to construction. This opportunity allows for real life testing of design solutions intended to enhance healing.

a joint venture

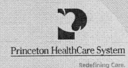

Princeton HealthCare System
Redefining Care.

Susan Lorenz, RN, DrNP (c), CNAA
VP Patient Care Services and Chief Nursing Officer, University Medical Center at Princeton

Ismini Naos, Senior Medical Planner, Hellmuth Obata + Kassabaum, PC

PURPOSE
The purpose of this poster presentation is to present the concept of designing a state of the art patient room using an evidence-based approach that assures that the environment is conducive to the healing of patients and promotion of wellness in staff.

1. The attendee will describe the components necessary to create a healing environment.

2. The attendee will identify specific design interventions that are intended to eliminate noise, provide optimal lighting and views, promote nursing presence, and provide for the safe care of patients.

3. The attendee will describe how the use of a functional mock up room will assist room designers and healthcare providers to assure that the patient room is a space where patients and families can cope with and transcend illness.

ABSTRACT
The design of the patient room is gaining increasing importance as evidence continues to be introduced that proves that the actual style of the room, along with the location of the furniture and amount of light and views that are part of the room may prevent adverse outcomes and hasten healing. The current hospital building boom has brought the research on patient rooms into the limelight and this emerging field continues to study the effect of room design on patients. Many new hospitals are sporting single patient rooms that are canted, same handed, and allow space for significant others to participate in the care of their loved ones.

At the University Medical Center at Princeton the new state of the art health care facility scheduled to open in 2011, a multidisciplinary team of hospital administrators, architects, medical planners and clinicians are working diligently to design a patient room that promotes efficiency in care delivery, provides ease of use for clinicians, maintains satisfied patients, reduces the occurrences of medical errors and allows for healing. This is a tall order and not one that is being taken lightly. In order to test principles of evidence based design and assure that the new patient room meets the expectations of both patients and staff, the design team in collaboration with hospital administration has proposed the building of a functional mock up room that will be in use in the current hospital for a minimum of 2 years prior to the opening of the new facility.

Source: University Medical Center at Princeton, Princeton, NJ. Used with permission.

References

1. Lankford M. G., et al.: *Limiting the Spread of Infection in Health Care Environments.* The Center for Health Design CHER Research Committee, Apr. 2007.

2. Hota S.: Outbreak of multidrug-resistant pseudomonas aeruginosa colonization and infection secondary to imperfect intensive care unit room design. http://www.journals.uchicago.edu/doi/abs/10.1086/592700?prevSearch=%28gardam%29+AND+%5Bjournal%3A+iche%5D (accessed Jun. 12, 2009).

Case Study 8-2: Getting to the Root of Infection Prevention and Control in the Environment of Care

A health care organization need not wait for a sentinel or adverse event report to undertake a systems-based quality improvement initiative. Determining whether a patient's death or injury was unanticipated is generally based on the patient's condition at the time of admission. For example, an otherwise healthy patient who is admitted for an elective procedure, develops a wound infection, becomes septic, and dies should be considered a sentinel event. A death or major permanent loss of function is considered a sentinel event if the outcome was not the result of the natural course of the patient's illness or underlying condition(s) that existed at the time of admission. Cases in which a patient is immunocompromised or has multiple comorbidities are more difficult to classify. In the absence of any infection outbreak, sentinel event, or unusually high rate of infection, staff at North Shore University Hospital in Manhasset, New York, undertook to reduce infection risk to immunocompromised patients. Explaining the reasoning behind the study, Joseph S. Cervia, M.D., F.A.C.P., F.A.A.P., clinical professor of medicine and pediatrics at the Albert Einstein College of Medicine (affiliated with North Shore University Hospital), states

that health care–associated infections (HAIs) are no longer considered an inevitable consequence of hospitalization, and in many cases are preventable.

Background

Through literature review, staff were aware that HAIs could be linked to hospital water, and that in the setting of outbreaks of known waterborne pathogens, water filtration had made substantial contributions to reduction in risk of these infections.[1] This study was not prompted by any sentinel event or unusually high infection rate, but was a proactive and multidisciplinary approach to preventing infection in high-risk patients.

Infections with gram-negative bacteria (GNB) such as *Pseudomonas aeruginosa* and *Stenotrophomonas maltophilia* are known to contribute to morbidity and mortality in hospitalized patients, particularly among immunocompromised patients like recipients of bone marrow transplants. Because infections with GNB are on the rise and are increasingly resistant to antimicrobial therapy, and despite the lack of any recognized outbreak, staff sought to determine whether water filtration at the point of use would result in a decreased infection risk among hospitalized bone marrow transplant patients.[2]

The primary goal of the initiative was to demonstrate whether a reduction in infection risk was possible. Understanding that bone marrow transplant patients are immunocompromised, and that one of the principle infection risks—GNB—is frequently culturable from health care water, Dr. Cervia hypothesized that a significant impact could be made on baseline infection rates by using a novel intervention directed at a perceived risk for this population.

Assembling a Team to Address the Problem

A multidisciplinary team was assembled including staff from the bone marrow transplant unit, infection prevention and control (IC), infectious disease, quality management, and facilities management. Frontline staff and individuals with diverse systems and process knowledge were included. The team defined, studied, and

Organization Facts

North Shore University Hospital is a tertiary-care facility and an academic campus for the New York University School of Medicine. The hospital has 731 beds and a staff of approximately 2,700 physicians.

Project Description

Based on voluntarily recorded data on infection rates, the Albert Einstein School of Medicine sought to reduce infection risk in immunocompromised patients in the bone marrow transplant unit, a 100%-occupied 4-bed unit. North Shore University Hospital staff examined whether infection risk could be impacted in the absence of recognized outbreak.

Outcomes

Clinical infection rates in the unit were reduced and zero infections were noted in eight months.

(continued on next page)

Case Study 8-2: *continued*

determined the problem (in this case, the presence of GNB infections in the bone marrow transplant unit), identifying contributing process factors and analyzing current systems to determine where redesign might reduce risk. The team brainstormed appropriate effectiveness of interventions, with an emphasis on ensuring that all appropriate IC interventions were already in place, and maintaining all current and appropriate IC practices, including hand hygiene, isolation precautions, and so forth.

Staff could reasonably conclude that from a systems-based approach, patient exposure to GNB in a bone marrow transplant unit would be expected to occur at some point due to ingestion, respiratory aerosols, and/or touch contact. Although patients may become colonized previous to admittance to the bone marrow transplant unit, bringing in the GNB in gut flora, it was agreed that it is far more common for patients to become immunocompromised first and then be exposed to gram-negative rods within the hospital. Since many pathogens in immunocompromised hosts have been associated with water, an intervention that precluded entry of these organisms into the point of use would be appropriate to try.

Methods
Unfiltered water was sampled from taps in the bone marrow transplant unit of a major U.S. teaching hospital and cultured at a reference laboratory. Water filters (specially adapted 0.2 micron filters) were installed at the point of use, including sinks, showers, and ice machines throughout the bone marrow transplant unit. Filters were replaced every 14 days per use instructions, and follow-up water cultures were performed. Data were collected on patients who experienced infection during the study period and were saved for analysis. Infection rates in the unit were tracked over a nine-month period and were compared

with the control period occurring just prior to point-of-use filtration.[2]

Staff Support
The trial was necessarily nonblinded. Staff were instructed not to change any IC processes, as any extraneous interventions might confound the ability to interpret results of the point-of-use filtration intervention. After point-of-use filters had been in place for three or four months, the infectious disease team already noticed there was a fall-off in consultations in the bone marrow transplant unit. Nurses in the bone marrow transplant unit also noted they were not seeing any infections in patients. Because of frontline staff experience of the fall-off in infections, support for point-of-use filtration was strong.

Results
The results of this initiative were highly statistically significant. Unfiltered water samples from 25% of taps cultured in the bone marrow transplant unit grew *Pseudomonas aeruginosa* and *Stenotrophomonas maltophilia*. Clinical infection rates in the unit were reduced from 50% in the period prior to point-of-use filtration to 6% ($p = 0.02$) in the nine-month period for which filters were in place. Zero infections were noted in eight of those nine months. The infections that did occur were *Staphylococcus* and *E. coli*, non-waterborne organisms.

Monitoring
Currently, staff are developing plans to test a similar change carefully, systematically, and unit by unit throughout the hospital. Late-stage plans have already been developed to introduce the initiative in the cardio-thoracic unit, where there are currently no other new interventions planned that might confound results. Staff continue to monitor vigilantly infection rates hospitalwide, particularly focused in areas where patients are immunocompromised.

(continued on next page)

Case Study 8-2: *continued*

Figure 1: Infection Rates in the Bone Marrow Transplant Unit (BMTU)

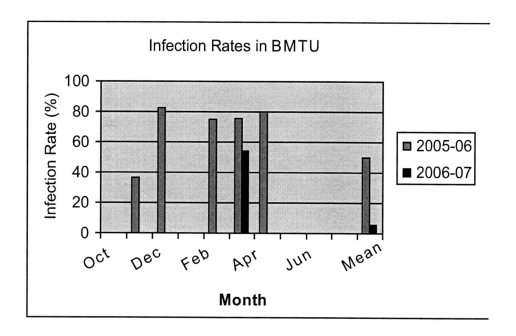

References:

1. Anaissie E.J., et al.: The hospital water supply as a source of nosocomial infections/A plea for action. *Arch Intern Med* 162:1483–1492, 2002.

2. Cervia J., et al.: Hospital water: A possible source of healthcare-associated infections in bone marrow transplant recipients [abstract]. Oral Symposium Presentation at the American Federation for Medical Research 2008 Eastern Regional Meeting, Washington, D.C., Apr. 9, 2008.

Typically done once a quarter or even once a year, this approach can help staff spot problems that might be missed on regular rounding.

How do you know which indicators to look for on either a regular or occasional basis? As with PI activity in other areas, organizations should look first to high-volume, high-risk, and problem-prone activities, populations, units, and sites. For example, a procedure that has been associated with a cluster of infections in the past would make a good target for continuous monitoring, as would a hallway that has experienced leakages or a sink that tends to attract

storage items underneath it. In addition, organizations often base indicators on new guidelines, procedures, or equipment—for example, is a new disinfectant being diluted properly?

Reports of employee injuries, illnesses, and exposures to potentially infectious material may be an indicator of an environmental issue. If there are cases of foodborne illness in employees, both the food and the equipment should be tested for organisms, temperature, preparation practices, and other practices. Table 8-1, page 128, provides a sample check sheet for employee injury reports.

- Another excellent way to identify problems or potential problems that could benefit from performance measurement and improvement activity is to interview employees. Do they know how to report incidents of exposure? Do they know where to find gloves, gowns, masks, and other items of PPE? If they come across a leak or a spill, do they know who to contact—or do they just clean it up themselves to save time?

Whether observing, interviewing, or rounding, the old adage applies: If you are going to ask the question, know what you are going to do with the answer. Unsatisfactory performance requires corrective action. It might be to revise a procedure, implement additional training, clarify signs, add checklists, alter staffing patterns, purchase new equipment, or even renovate a building. Whatever the action, it should be documented and followed up: Was it done? when? by whom? What were the results? If the actions didn't achieve the desired effects, then it is time to re-examine the evidence and rethink the approach.

In short, the tried and true method using a plan-do-check-act (PDCA) cycle of improvement, in which the organization identifies a process—ideally, a single step or element in a process—for improvement, implements a solution, and monitors the effectiveness of the solution on an ongoing basis, is applicable to these situations.

Whether good or bad, the results of performance measurement and improvement should be shared with all staff who will be involved, even tangentially, in data collection and implementation efforts. Such staff will probably include direct caregivers, support staff, and supervisors. They need to know exactly what to collect and, just as important, why they are collecting it. What is the goal? How will it help them and their colleagues provide better service? Relate the organization's infection rates back to the job each staff

member is doing and to their common goals. In short, center educational efforts on the practical applications for processes that individuals do during the performance of their jobs and align them with the organization's mission.

Using Data Tools to Improve the Infection Prevention and Control Program

PI activities use a variety of statistical and nonstatistical tools in the continuous cycle of collecting and evaluating data as organizations look for opportunities to improve and revise systems. Some tools are used to collect and analyze data, whereas others generate ideas, determine the root cause of a problem, or help people understand a process. It is easy to become buried in data collection and evaluation and overlook analysis and action. To prevent this situation, organizations need to know which tool to use for what purpose. Table 8-2, page 129, lists a number of common PI tools and their uses.

Employees who are not competent to carry them out can undermine even the most effective policies and procedures. This point is as true for the people who maintain medical equipment or utility systems as it is for direct caregivers. For this reason, the Joint Commission requires that accredited organizations assess each person's knowledge, skills, behavior, and abilities to perform his or her job at hire or application, after orientation, whenever new services or technology is introduced, and at regular intervals set by leadership.

The point of this exercise is to identify persons and areas needing improvement to develop and schedule appropriate and effective education and training programs. If, for example, a significant number of maintenance workers are not using PPE properly—if they do not know where it is kept or cannot demonstrate the right way to put it on—then this aspect of IC training needs reinforcement.

Table 8-1: Sample Check Sheet: Employee Injury Reports: Frequency Over Six Months							
Causes	*Jan*	*Feb*	*Mar*	*Apr*	*May*	*Jun*	*Total*
Sharps	*1*	*3*	*4*	*1*	*0*	*2*	*11*
Falls	*3*	*2*	*0*	*3*	*1*	*2*	*11*
Violence	*1*	*1*	*1*	*0*	*2*	*1*	*6*
Maintenance accidents	*1*	*4*	*0*	*2*	*1*	*3*	*11*
Monthly Total	*6*	*10*	*5*	*6*	*4*	*8*	——
This sample check sheet illustrates common causes of employee injuries.							

Organizations that can pinpoint where educational efforts are needed have a better chance of having leadership allocate adequate resources for the task; this process means collecting, aggregating, and analyzing competence assessment data. Sidebar 8-1, page 130, presents a formula for putting data into action.

A histogram is a bar graph that displays the variation in a set of repeated measurements over time. It is used to analyze a process to determine whether consistent, positive results can be achieved or improved. One use of this tool in PI is to measure the effects of training in one or another aspect of IC. Figure 8-1, page 130, shows how this tool can be used to determine how many employees need additional education in infection transmission routes following annual IC training.

One way to look at the durability of training over time is to use a sample run chart. Also called line graphs, run charts are used to identify problems and trends within a process over time and are especially useful for monitoring performance during the check step of the PDCA cycle. For example, if an organization wanted to determine the effectiveness of its training in decontamination procedures after switching from printed illustrations to videotape, it might construct a run chart similar to the one shown in Figure 8-2, page 131.

The CDC's Guidelines for Environmental Infection Control in Health-Care Facilities offer a great deal of helpful information to both IC and EC professionals. However, given that infections caused by microorganisms described in the guideline are rare events, and that the effect of the recommendations on infection rates in a facility might not be readily measurable, the CDC suggests that organizations evaluate the recommendations using five steps to measure performance, as outlined in Sidebar 8-2, page 131. The same five steps could be used to determine the effectiveness of an organization's overall IC program.

Table 8-2: Performance Improvement Tool Selection Matrix

Tool	Measurement	Analysis	Action	Review
Flowchart	X	X	X	
Cause-and-effect diagram	X	X		
Brainstorming	X	X	X	X
PDCA	X	X	X	X
Line graph or run chart	X		X	X
Histogram		X		X
Pareto chart	X	X		X
Scatter diagram		X		X
Control chart	X	X	X	
Check sheet		X		
Decision matrix	X		X	
These are not the only PI tools available to health care organizations, of course, but they are among the most commonly used.				

Sidebar 8-1: Numerators, Denominators, and Target Rates

So you collected the data: What do you do with it? Using a hypothetical example, say an organization collects data indicating that only 40% of employees are complying with hand hygiene protocols. It institutes a more rigorous training regimen, posts reminder signs on every unit, and puts the issue on the agenda at all departmental meetings. The result of these activities is a jump in compliance—all the way to 55%. Still a long way from an idealistic goal, or is this effort "good enough?" Will the increase hold over time? The only way to know is to measure again and again.

But what is "good enough?" Few processes involving human beings operate at 100%. Although it might be realistic to aim for 100% in terms of numbers of employees who get an annual skin test for tuberculosis, say, it is not realistic to expect 100% of employees to wash their hands 100% of the time.

To track performance, trend variance, measure statistical significance, and calculate an acceptable target rate, an organization must first establish realistic baseline rates.

A target might be a single number or a range, based on past performance, expert opinion or consensus, published research, internal or external benchmarks, or best practices described in the literature or by professional organizations. For example, you might aim at having 95% of housekeeping and laundry employees use standard precautions, as measured by periodic observation.

A measurement might be a rate, a percentage, or a ratio, but to be useful, it must be constructed appropriately. If a hospital is monitoring the timely emptying of sharps containers, the denominator will be all the sharps containers in the facility (say 400), and they may select as a numerator those containers that were found to be more than three-quarters full. A numerator of 40, then, would mean that 10% (40/400) of containers were not being emptied per policy, compared with perhaps 2% allowed by the organization's own standard. After the organization implements a plan of action, continued monitoring would indicate whether further improvement efforts were required.

Figure 8-1: Sample Histogram: Post-test Scores for Infection Transmission Education

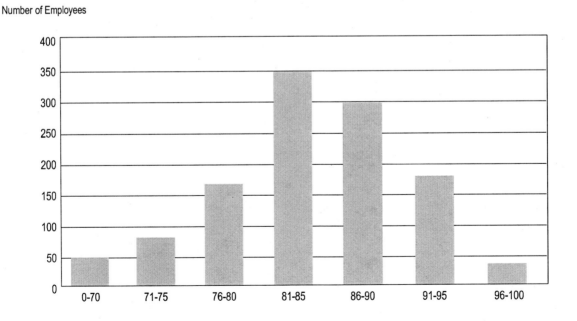

Number of Employees

The fact that 325 of 1160 employees failed to make a passing grade (81) suggests that training methods need revision.

Figure 8-2: Sample Run Chart: Effectiveness of Training in Decontamination Procedures

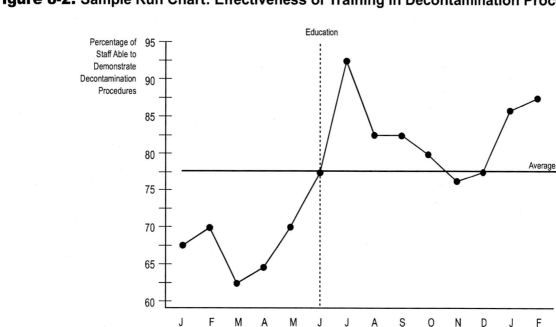

These data show that employees are clearest on decontamination procedures in the month following training and that the effects of traning remain relatively strong six months later.

Sidebar 8-2: Centers for Disease Control and Prevention Recommendations for Measuring Infection Prevention and Control (IC) Efforts

- Document whether IC personnel are actively involved in all phases of a health care facility's demolition, construction, and renovation. Activities should include performing a risk assessment of the necessary types of construction barriers and daily monitoring and documenting of the presence of negative airflow within the construction zone or renovation area.

- Monitor and document daily the negative airflow in airborne infection isolation (AII) rooms and the positive airflow in protective environment (PE) rooms, especially when patients are in these rooms.

- Perform assays at least once a month by using standard quantitative methods for endotoxin in water used to reprocess hemodialyzers and for heterotrophic and mesophilic bacteria in water used to prepared dialysate and for hemodialyzer reprocessing.

- Evaluate possible environmental sources (for example, water, lab solutions, or reagents) of specimen contamination when nontuberculous mycobacteria (NTM) of unlikely clinical importance are isolated from clinical cultures. If environmental contamination is found, eliminate the probable mechanisms.

- Document policies to identify and respond to water damage. Such policies should result in either repair or drying of wet structural or porous materials within 72 hours or removal of the wet material if drying is unlikely within 72 hours.

Source: McKibben L., et al.: Guidance on Public Reporting of Healthcare-Associated Infections: Recommendations of the Healthcare Infection Control Practices Advisory Committee, *Am J Infect Control* 33, May 2005. http://www.cdc.gov/ncidod/hip/PublicReportingGuide.pdf (accessed Feb. 19, 2009).

Conclusion

Careful attention to every detail in an organization's physical environment is the best and only path toward lower infection risks and mitigating infections when they do happen. Monitoring those details is a true team effort, from leaders to frontline and supporting staff. With the proper policies and procedures implemented, and by analyzing human factor topics, equipment, environmental services, utilities, construction and renovation, emergency management, and practicing performance measurement and improvement, IC in the EC can be preserved all day, every day, in every health care organization.

Index

A

AAMI (Association for the Advancement of Medical Instrumentation), 38

AIA. *See* American Institute of Architects (AIA)

Airborne contaminants. *See also Aspergillus* species and aspergillosis
- construction and renovation and, 85, 86, 94, 102
- control of, 65
- examples of, 65
- HAI prevention, viii, 8
- prevention of, 7
- sick-building syndrome (SBS), 68, 72–73
- UVGI and, 66

Airborne infection isolation (AII) rooms, 68, 84, 94

Airborne precautions, 51

Air conditioning system. *See* Heating, ventilation, and air conditioning (HVAC) systems

Air embolism, vii

Air exchange rates, 66, 67–68, 94, 101, 108

Air pressure relationships, 66–67

Air quality maintenance checklist, 71

Alcohol-based hand rubs and dispensers, 19, 22–23, 27

Allegheny County (Pennsylvania) Health Department, 79

Ambulatory care organization decontamination activities, 108, 110

American Gastroenterological Association, 38

American Institute of Architects (AIA)
- air pressure relationships, 67
- construction and renovation guidelines, 84, 87
- facility design recommendations, 83, 84
- *Guidelines for Design and Construction of Hospital and Health Care Facilities*, 66, 83, 87
- HEPA filters, 67
- HVAC system design, 65–66, 67
- infection control risk assessments (ICRAs), 83
- regulations and guidelines from, 65–66
- tap-water temperature recommendations, 75
- ventilation rate requirements, 68

American National Standards Institute (ANSI), 73

American Society for Healthcare Engineering (ASHE), 22, 83

American Society of Heating, Refrigerating and Air Conditioning Engineers (ASHRAE)
- *Handbook—HVAC Applications* (ASHRAE), 66, 87
- *HVAC Design Manual for Hospitals and Clinics*, 66
- HVAC system design, 65–66
- regulations and guidelines from, 65–66
- ventilation rate requirements, 68

ANSI (American National Standards Institute), 73

Anthrax exposure, 109

AORN (Association of periOperative Registered Nurses), 38, 43, 46

APIC. *See* Association for Professionals in Infection Control and Epidemiology (APIC)

ASHE (American Society for Healthcare Engineering), 22, 83

ASHRAE. *See* American Society of Heating, Refrigerating and Air Conditioning Engineers (ASHRAE)

Aspergillus species and aspergillosis
- case study, 95–98
- characteristics of, 65
- construction and renovation and, 86, 102
- control of, 65
- threat from, viii, 8, 65
- water distribution system, disease outbreaks traced to, 73

Association for Professionals in Infection Control and Epidemiology (APIC)
- alcohol-based hand rubs and dispenser recommendations, 22
- biomedical engineering, 43
- equipment cleaning strategies, 38, 43
- Hand Hygiene Task Force, 18
- regulation and guideline resources, 87

Association for the Advancement of Medical Instrumentation (AAMI), 38

Association of periOperative Registered Nurses (AORN), 38, 43, 46

B

Bar graph, 129, 130

Biological indicators (BI), 38

Biomedical engineering, 39, 43

Blood and other potentially infectious materials
- Bloodborne Pathogen Standard (OSHA), 27–28, 30, 51, 52, 60
- central nervous system (CNS) precautions, 45–46, 47
- decontamination of surfaces in contact with, 51, 52
- disposal of, 60, 61
- exposure to, 8

Bloodborne Pathogen Standard (OSHA), 27–28, 30, 51, 52, 60

Blood incompatibility, costs associated with, vii

Bloodstream infections
- central line–associated bloodstream infections (CLABSI), 8, 13
- costs associated with, CMS reimbursements for, vii
- medical equipment and devices and, 8
- National Patient Safety Goal 7, 8
- prevention of, 8